Dermatology - Laboratory and Clinical Research

Acne

Etiology, Treatment Options and Social Effects

DERMATOLOGY - LABORATORY AND CLINICAL RESEARCH

Additional books in this series can be found on Nova's website
under the Series tab.

Additional e-books in this series can be found on Nova's website
under the e-book tab.

DERMATOLOGY - LABORATORY AND CLINICAL RESEARCH

ACNE

ETIOLOGY, TREATMENT OPTIONS AND SOCIAL EFFECTS

MOHAMED L. ELSAIE
EDITOR

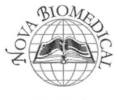

New York

Copyright © 2013 by Nova Science Publishers, Inc.

All rights reserved. No part of this book may be reproduced, stored in a retrieval system or transmitted in any form or by any means: electronic, electrostatic, magnetic, tape, mechanical photocopying, recording or otherwise without the written permission of the Publisher.

For permission to use material from this book please contact us:
Telephone 631-231-7269; Fax 631-231-8175
Web Site: http://www.novapublishers.com

NOTICE TO THE READER

The Publisher has taken reasonable care in the preparation of this book, but makes no expressed or implied warranty of any kind and assumes no responsibility for any errors or omissions. No liability is assumed for incidental or consequential damages in connection with or arising out of information contained in this book. The Publisher shall not be liable for any special, consequential, or exemplary damages resulting, in whole or in part, from the readers' use of, or reliance upon, this material. Any parts of this book based on government reports are so indicated and copyright is claimed for those parts to the extent applicable to compilations of such works.

Independent verification should be sought for any data, advice or recommendations contained in this book. In addition, no responsibility is assumed by the publisher for any injury and/or damage to persons or property arising from any methods, products, instructions, ideas or otherwise contained in this publication.

This publication is designed to provide accurate and authoritative information with regard to the subject matter covered herein. It is sold with the clear understanding that the Publisher is not engaged in rendering legal or any other professional services. If legal or any other expert assistance is required, the services of a competent person should be sought. FROM A DECLARATION OF PARTICIPANTS JOINTLY ADOPTED BY A COMMITTEE OF THE AMERICAN BAR ASSOCIATION AND A COMMITTEE OF PUBLISHERS.

Additional color graphics may be available in the e-book version of this book.

Library of Congress Cataloging-in-Publication Data

ISBN: 978-1-62618-358-2

Library of Congress Control Number:2013933806

Published by Nova Science Publishers, Inc. † *New York*

Contents

Preface		vii
Chapter I	Acne: A Review on Epidemiology, Pathogenesis and Treatment Options *Richa Sharma and Namrita Lall*	1
Chapter II	Acne: Pathogenesis, Therapy and Social Effects *Gabriella Fabbrocini, Sara Cacciapuoti, Dario Bianca and Giuseppe Monfrecola*	15
Chapter III	Selected Thai Medicinal Plant for the Treatment of Acne: Garciniamangostana Linn *Panupon Khumsupan and Wandee Gritsanapan*	41
Chapter IV	Acne and IGF-I: A Fascinating Hypothesis *Elena Guanziroli, Laura Maffeis and Mauro Barbareschi*	69
Chapter V	Melanocortin-1 and -5 Receptors as Targets for Acne Therapy *Wen-Hwa Li, Li Zhang and Miri Seiberg*	89
Chapter VI	Psychosocial and Emotional Aspects of Acne: The Need for a Psychosomatic Approach to Management *K. Stephen and A. G. Affleck*	107

Chapter VII	Light Cautery in the Treatment of Closed Comedones *V. Bettoli, S. Zauli and A. Virgili*	**147**
Index		**153**

Preface

Although many dermatological diseases are not life threatening, they pose a unique challenge to the human psyche. Cutaneous disease carries a distinctive psychosocial burden in that patients who suffer from these diseases are often unable to hide their condition from public scrutiny. Specifically, acne vulgaris is a ubiquitous disease with a known potential to cause significant psychological repercussions. Acne is the leading cause for visits to a dermatologist and affects more than 80 percent of adolescents. Acne can affect up to 50.9 percent of women and 42.5 percent of men throughout their 20s and can continue to occur throughout adulthood. Between 30 to 50 percent of adolescents experience psychological difficulties associated with acne, including body image concerns, embarrassment, social impairment, anxiety, frustration, anger, depression, and poor self-esteem. Additionally, suicidal ideation and suicide attempts related to the negative psychosocial impacts of acne have also been documented. Not only does acne result in emotional distress, the anxiety evoked by having acne can aggravate the skin condition itself, thereby creating a vicious cycle. Acne is the most common problem that presents to dermatologists. Although acne does not cause direct physical impairment, it can produce a significant psychosocial burden. Acne commonly involves the face. Facial appearance represents an important aspect of one's perception of body image. Therefore, it is not surprising that a susceptible individual with facial acne may develop significant psychosocial disability. As part of the emotional impact, increased levels of anxiety, anger, depression, and frustration are observed in patients with acne. Acne's consequences can prove very traumatic for adolescent patients. This suggests that the impact of acne can be more serious for the patients than most clinicians think it would be and it is more important to focus on the subjective perception in managing acne patients, irrespective of the objective severity. Our book highlights and tackles several aspects of acne and magnifies the importance of screening for psychosocial problems in those who present for management of acne. It is important for all health service workers to be cautious about psychological morbidity in young people, and especially dermatologists should be aware of the importance of basic psychosomatic treatment in conjunction with medical treatment in the management of acne.

Chapter I – Acne is a general name given to a skin disorder in which the sebaceous glands become inflamed and is one of the most common diseases of the skin. It is more prevalent in boys in adolescence but women are more affected during adulthood. *Propionibacterium acnes*, the causative agent plays a pivot role in the etiology. Brief anatomy and morphology of *P. acnes* with help of transmission electron micrographs are explained. The review provides pathogenesis and immunology of acne. *P. acnes* induce monocytes to secrete pro-inflammatory cytokines like interleukins (IL-8, IL-1β) and tumor necrosis factor (TNFα) and thus play an important role in pathogenesis of inflammatory acne. Conventional drugs for treating acne are discussed along with possible side effects. The plant kingdom is known to contain many novel biologically active compounds, many of which could potentially have a higher medicinal value when compared to some of the current medications. The new era of traditional medicine and cosmeceutical with an emphasis on plant derived drugs as an alternative treatment option are explained.

Chapter II – Acne vulgaris is a common skin condition with substantial cutaneous and psychologic disease burden. The emotional impact of acne is comparable to that experienced by patients with systemic diseases, like diabetes and epilepsy. Its pathophysiology is multifactorial and complex, including obstruction of the pilosebaceous unit due to increased sebum production, abnormal keratinization, proliferation of Propionibacterium acnes and inflammation. Topical agents (retinoids, benzoyl peroxide and antibacterials) are the most commonly used therapy for acne. Newer topical therapy, such as photodynamic therapy, has been proposed to increase efficacy when conventional therapies are ineffective. This chapter discusses the etiology, pathogenesis, treatment and psychological impact of acne vulgaris.

Chapter III – Acne vulgaris is a skin disease occurring at the cutaneous layer. It is characterized by inflammatory or non-inflammatory lesions due to the overproduction and blockage of sebum and keratinous debris in sebaceous follicles. This accumulation acts as a precursor of acne lesions called microcomedo and is highly susceptible to bacterial infection, namely *Propionibacterium acnes* and *Staphylococcus epidermidis*. Many Thai traditional herbal medicines have been recognized as effective acne treatment, including turmeric (*Curcuma longa* Linn.), Centella (*Centellaasiatica* (L.)Urb.), *Chromolaenaodorata*(L.) R. M. King and H. Rob., *Houttuyniacordata* Thunb., *Sennaalata* (L.) Roxb., *Melaleucaalternifolia* (Maiden and Betche) Cheel.,and mangosteen (*Garciniamangostana* Linn.). Searching for an alternative treatment has been a paramount focus in the medical field due to antibiotic resistance. Traditional medicine also has its advantage of lower side effects and abundant availability. Many traditional medicines have been under intense scrutiny for such purpose and one of the most effective herbs is mangosteen. Many researchers have reported its antimicrobial property, especially against*P. acnes* and *S. epidermidis*, and its anti-inflammatory and antioxidant properties. Due to these combinatorial properties, mangosteen and many herbal medicines with similar properties would be effective candidates to the treatment of acne. Mangosteen or *Garciniamangostana* Linn.of the family Guttiferae is one of the most consumed fruits and distributed widely in the countries in the tropical zone. Because of its sweet and delicious taste, it is the economic fruit especially of the countries in the South East Asia. Many chemical compounds in mangosteen are responsible for its medicinal properties and the one that is present in the highest amount is α-mangostin, extracted from the rind and is especially abundant in the ripe rind. Mangosteen extract has been more popularly utilized in the cosmetic industries due to the fact that it is able to inhibit acne causing bacteria including *P. acnes* (MIC 7.81μg/mL and MBC 31.25μg/mL) and *S. epidermidis* (MIC 15.63μg/mL and MBC 31.25μg/mL). Many other xanthones, tannins and phenols, which contribute to the antioxidant and anti-inflammatory activities, can alsobe found in mangosteen.

Chapter IV – Acne vulgaris is a common chronic inflammatory disease that affects the pilosebaceous follicle. Its pathophysiology is complex and multifactorial, with strong evidence supporting the involvement of increased sebum production, abnormal differentiation of skin keratinocytes, bacterial colonization, and inflammation. Recent experimental studies have suggested that acne is influenced by insulin/ insulin-like growth factor-1 (IGF-1) – signalling and may be considered an IGF-1-mediated disease. The purpose of this review article consists in delineating the role of insulin/ IGF-1 pathway in the pathogenesis of acne, its relationship with androgen hormones and the possible pharmacological and dietary intervention in restoring its equilibrium. The IGF-1 activity rises during puberty by the action of increased GH secretion and is amplified by insulin, which inhibits the production of IGF binding protein-1 (IGFBP-1). Diets rich in carbohydrates with a high glycaemic index, which are associated with hyperglycaemia and reactive hyperinsulinaemia, increase formation of IGF-1. In addition to this, the *P. acnes,* which alone is able to activate the keratinocyte IGF-1/IGF-1 receptor system has also a central role in comedogenesis. IGF-1 promotes and maintains the expression of steroidogenic enzymes that are responsible for converting cholesterol into steroid precursors for the synthesis of dehydroepiandrosterone (DHEA) and androgens. Steroidogenic enzymes are expressed in human sebaceous glands where they may stimulate local androgen production. Moreover, IGF-1 can induce 5alpha-reductase in human skin fibroblasts, leading to an increased conversion of testosterone to dihydrotestosterone (DHT). It has recently been demonstrated that IGF-1 can increase lipid production in sebocytes *in vitro* via the activation of IGF-1 receptor through multiple pathways. Clinically, significantly higher IGF-1 levels have been described in women with acne compared with control subjects. The number of total acne lesions, inflammatory lesions, and serum levels of DHT are related with serum IGF-1 levels in women with acne. A correlation between the mean facial sebum excretion rate and serum IGF-1 levels has been shown in postadolescent acne patients. Pharmacological down-regulation of insulin/ IGF-1 signaling has been demonstrated with metformin, oral isotretinoin, and zinc treatment. These are promising options for the treatment of acne vulgaris, and conditions with insulin resistence, and increased IGF-1 serum levels. Patients with persistent acne, and with endocrine disorders, especially those with genetic variations of the IGF1 gene expressing increased IGF-1 serum levels, may benefit from dietary modifications including a reduction of dairy and hyperglycaemic foods.

Chapter V – Excessive sebum production is a key to the pathology of acne vulgaris, and the inhibition of sebum secretion predicts acne therapy outcome. Effective treatments for acne, such as isotretinoin and androgen modulators, inhibit sebaceous gland differentiation and sebum production. However, these agents also induce undesired effects, which limit their use in the clinics. Melanocortins, a series of neuropeptides derived from a parent pro-opiomelanocortin (POMC) molecule, bind to the melanocortin receptors. The melanocortin receptors 1 and 5 (MC1R, MC5R) are expressed in the sebaceous glands. MC1R has been associated with acne lesions, and MC5R is a marker of differentiated sebocytes. The production of sebaceous lipids is impaired in MC5R deficient mice, suggesting that MC5R is a regulator of sebum production. Therefore, the sebaceous gland melanocortin receptors were investigated as possible targets for acne therapy. A dual MC1R and MC5R antagonist was shown to inhibit sebocyte differentiation in primary human sebocyte cultures, and to reduce sebum production in human skins transplanted onto immuno-deficient mice. These studies suggest that dual MC1R and MC5R antagonists may serve as potential topical therapeutic agents for sebaceous disorders with excess sebum, such as acne.

Chapter VI – Acne usually presents in adolescents, a time of physical change and emotional instability. This extra change in self-image can compromise self-esteem and self-consciousness further. In individuals with extra risk factors and reduced resilience factors, the coping mechanism can be tipped out of balance leading to psychological and functional morbidity. It has long been recognised that in some people with acne, stress appears to contribute towards flare ups. Such stress-responders may benefit from relaxation training and other aspects of stress management. There is a spectrum of emotional sequelae secondary to acne: some individuals appear to be extremely stoical and resistant to emotional morbidity with positive coping mechanisms, even with objectively severe acne on physical examination; other individuals appear to be more prone to emotional morbidity even when objectively there is mild acne; the reasons for this are complex and have been addressed in several studies. Unfavourable coping is found in 5 associated psychiatric disorders, namely:adjustment disorder, depression, social phobia and anxiety disorder. eating disorder and Body Dysmorphic Disorder. Therefore, it is best practice to assess patients who have acne for such associated psychological comorbidities to achieve maximum benefit and minimise risk to the patient. When psychiatric comorbidity is present, it should be addressed and treated and when necessary, referral to a specialist in mental health is desirable. A psychosomatic approach to a new patient with acne based on the biopsychosocial model of illness is desirable. Further assessment and treatment is individualised to that patient. Simple measures like use of SUbjective Discomfort Scores (SUDS), self reported by the patient, assessing general well being, anxiety, depression and stress are a good starting point. Core communication skills and basic counselling to generate a strong rapport with the patient, demonstrating empathy and exploring the impact on quality of life and the patients perceived ideas and illness perception is useful. Most patients with acne do not have severe associated psychological morbidity and one needs to avoid "psychologicalising" them, but a minority do and these are the at-risk patients that we need to identify, as unfortunately suicide is a recognised association in such patients. The use of validated general health questionnaires, mental health questionnaires and dermatology-specific questionnaires can also help in information gathering. Acne excoriee can be helped with a combined therapeutic approach including behavioural therapy habit reversal training. Time is a limiting factor in busy clinics, however efforts should be made to allow for more time for individual patients who have unmet needs, and a multidisciplinary approach using perhaps an experienced nurse to listen to, and talk with appropriate patients in a counselling capacity or indeed referral to colleagues in Clinical Psychology or liaison Psychiatry when necessary. A motivated, trained and knowledgeable Dermatologist can help patients who have acne and significant psychosocial detriment with a well thought out, planned, holistic approach using conventional topical therapy, oral therapy, including isotretinoin, and psychological therapy whether it be supportive, motivational or cognitive-behavioural and occasionally psychopharmacological therapy. This psychosomatic approach will result in better patient outcome with increased patient satisfaction.

Chapter VII – Closed comedones are non inflammatory acne lesions which frequently precede inflammatory acne lesions. They consist on depositions of sebum surrounded by layers of horny cells and they can persist for a long time unless they are treated. Persistence of closed comedones may be responsible for reduced response to acne treatments and flare-up of inflammatory acne during oral isotretinoin assumption. Moreover, closed comedones, if not properly treated, are responsible for psychological distress in patients with acne; therefore their treatment is fundamental to improve quality of life. Topical and systemic retinoids are the mainstay of their medical treatment, but although used for long periods of time they can be unsuccessful. Therefore their extraction is a mandatory procedure to obtain full clearance of acne. Alternative treatments to eliminate closed comedones include cautery, surgery (physical extraction) and laser. Comparative studies matching different tecniques are not available in the literature. The authors describe the techniques of light cautery in the treatment of close comedones and compare efficacy and tolerability of this procedure with the other aforementioned treatments. Moreover they report their personal experience.

In: Acne
Editor: Mohamed L. Elsaie

ISBN: 978-1-62618-358-2
© 2013 Nova Science Publishers, Inc.

Chapter I

Acne: A Review on Epidemiology, Pathogenesis and Treatment Options

Richa Sharma and Namrita Lall
University of Pretoria

Abstract

Acne is a general name given to a skin disorder in which the sebaceous glands become inflamed and is one of the most common diseases of the skin. It is more prevalent in boys in adolescence but women are more affected during adulthood. *Propionibacterium acnes*, the causative agent plays a pivot role in the etiology. Brief anatomy and morphology of *P. acnes* with help of transmission electron micrographs are explained. The review provides pathogenesis and immunology of acne. *P. acnes* induce monocytes to secrete pro-inflammatory cytokines like interleukins (IL-8, IL-1β) and tumor necrosis factor (TNFα) and thus play an important role in pathogenesis of inflammatory acne. Conventional drugs for treating acne are discussed along with possible side effects. The plant kingdom is known to contain many novel biologically active compounds, many of which could potentially have a higher medicinal value when compared to some of the current medications. The new era of traditional medicine and cosmeceutical with an emphasis on plant derived drugs as an alternative treatment option are explained.

1. Introduction

Traditional medicine is almost as old as the existence of mankind. This statement is backed by evidence obtained from studies of human settlements of older civilizations. Paleontologists have found bunches of medicinal herbs among the fossilized remains (Normann and Snyman, 1996). Plants are the oldest source of medicine. People of almost all cultures have used them routinely. Before the modern pharmaceutical industry existed, people relied on folk knowledge and apothecaries (Spinella, 2005). To illustrate historical role of plant derived medicines, here are some well-known examples:

- Quinine- an alkaloid obtained from bark of *Cinchona pubescence*. Only effective remedy for malaria for more than 300 years.
- Atropine- alkaloid from *Atropa belladona*. Used as heart tonics, eye drops, and injected to treat Parkinsonism.
- Morphine, codine- alkaloid obtained from *Papaver sominiferum*. Morphine is powerful analgesic and codeine as headache remedy and ingredient of cough syrup.
- Taxol- diterpenoid from bark of *Taxus brevifolius*. Highly effective against cancer.
- Quassinoids- terpenoid from *Quassia amara*, is used to improve appetite and treat minor stomach ailments (Van Wyk et al., 1997).

Plants are of relevance to dermatology for both their adverse and beneficial effects on skin and skin disorders respectively. Virtually all cultures worldwide have relied historically, or continue to rely on medicinal plants for primary health care. Approximately one-third of all traditional medicines are for treatment of wounds or skin disorders, compared to only 1-3% of modern drugs.

The use of such medicinal plant extracts for the treatment of skin disorders arguably has been based largely on historical/anecdotal evidence. Beneficial aspects of medicinal plants on skin include: healing of wounds and burn injuries (especially *Aloe vera*); antifungal, antiviral, antibacterial and acaricidal activity against skin infections such as acne, herpes and scabies (especially tea tree (*Melaleuca alternifolia*) oil); activity against inflammatory/immune disorders affecting skin (e.g. psoriasis); and anti-tumour promoting activity against skin cancer (Mantle et al., 2001).

2. Cosmeceuticals

Cosmetics based on herbs and other botanicals are as old as civilization itself. Egypt, the cradle of one of the earliest ancient cultures, pioneered natural perfumes and skin care preparations. Bath oils and rubs, moisturizing and cleansing lotions for skin, shampoos and conditioners for hair, all these products utilize the oils and other by-products of herbs both as main ingredients and subtle additives (Hoffmann and Manning, 2002). Plant based cosmetics were also common in ancient Greece and in Roman Empire (Burlando et al., 2010). Plants have emerged as the best source of cosmetics ingredients that meet the consumer's growing demand of natural character, efficiency, safety, and are increasingly replacing synthetic ingredients. Nowadays, cosmetic ingredients are designed by producers, used by consumers and investigated by researchers to examine their potential for cosmeceutical development. In cosmetic lingo, there is a name given "cosmeceuticals" (Figure 1), that merges cosme(tic) and (pharma)ceutical implications. This term indicates cosmetic-pharmaceutical hybrids aimed at enhancing the beauty by means of ingredients that provide additional health-related function or benefit (Burlando et al., 2010).

3. Skin and Acne

Skin is the largest organ of the body. It serves many important functions, including protection, precutaneous absorption, temperature regulation, fluid maintenance, sensory and disease control (Gebelein, 1997). Skin complaints affects all ages from neonatal to elderly and cause harm in number of ways. It has been estimated that skin diseases account to as high as 34% of all occupational disease (Spiewak, 2000). Acne is an altered or inflammatory state of hair follicle and associated sebaceous glands, involving the formation of a plug of keratin and sebum (a microcomedo) which can grow to form an open comedo (blackhead) or closed comedo (whitehead). It is further worsen by *Propionibacterium acnes*, thus producing inflammatory lesions such as papules, pustules, or nodule (Burlando et al., 2010). *P. acnes* are gram-positive anaerobic bacteria that are a component of the normal microbiota of human skin. An increased secretion of sebum is accompanied by thickening of epidermis at the outlet to the pilosebaceous follicles. This creates an obstruction to flow, and a comedo develops.

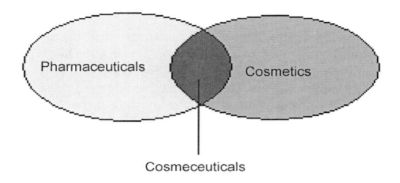

Figure 1. Cosmeceuticals.

Colonization of the follicle with *P. acnes* and the host inflammatory response to this plays a pivotal role in the development of the typical inflammatory papulopustular lesion (Shaw and Kennedy, 2007). It can range from occasional blemishes to a devastating, continuing episode leading to a permanent scaring.

It develops due to genetic predisposition during puberty. The years of greatest severity are from 16 to 19. The location of acne lesions is generally face, neck, back and chest (Williams and Schmitt, 1996). Several rating scales are developed with the aim of trying to grade the severity of acne. Below is classification to describe three grades of acne.

- Mild Acne

Patients with mild acne typically have predominantly open and closed comedones (blackheads and whiteheads) with a small number of active lesions normally confined to the face. Mild acne should not cause permanent scarring. Any or all of the following is present: small, tender, red papules; pustules; and blackheads and/or whiteheads. Mild acne is therefore characterized by the presence of a few to several papules and pustules, but no nodules.

- Moderate Acne

Similar to mild acne, but more papules and pustules. Patients with moderate acne typically have a few to several nodules. Lesions are often painful and there is a real possibility of scarring.

- Severe Acne

Similar to moderate acne but with nodular abscesses, leading to extensive scarring. Patients with severe acne have numerous or extensive lesions (Truter, 2009).

4. Epidemiology

Acne affects approximately 80% of people aged 11 to 30 years at some time, with about 60% of those sufficiently affected to seek treatment. Acne lesions typically develop at the onset of puberty. Girls therefore tend to develop acne at an earlier age than boys. The peak incidence for girls is between 14 and 17 years, compared with 15 to 19 years for boys. There may be a familial tendency to acne and it is slightly more common in boys, who also experience more severe involvement. Acne is more common in males than females during adolescence, but is more common in women than in men during adulthood. In addition, white patients are more likely to experience moderate to severe acne, although black skin is prone to worse scarring. Acne usually resolves within 10 years of onset, although up to five percent of women and one percent of men in their thirties can have mild persistent acne. The incidence of acne appears to have fallen in recent years, however the reasons are unknown (Truter, 2009).

Community-based studies in the UK, Australia, New Zealand, and Singapore have found prevalence rates ranging from 27% in early adolescence to 93% in late adolescence. The proportions of acne vulgaris in hospital-based studies of skin disease in Africa have been reported to be 4.6% in Ghana, 6.7% in Nigeria, and up to 17.5% in South Africa. Although, in a preliminary study of the dermatologic needs of a small rural community in Ethiopia, found that only three of 66 children (4.5%) between the ages of 10 and 16 years attending a school had acne, the knowledge of the prevalence and severity of acne in the larger community in Africa is very poor (Yahya, 2009). The first survey of dermatological disorders in South Africa was undertaken in 1957.In this study the relative frequency of skin disease in black patients was calculated as the percentage of dermatological outpatients. Out of 7029 dermatological outpatients, 1121 i.e. 16% were affected by acne from which 17.5 % were black, 7.3 % were white,13.9 % were coloured and 13.4 %were Indian (Hartshorne, 2003).

5. Propionibacterium Acnes, the Causative Agent

Propionibacterium acnes are pleomorphic, coryneform anaerobic Gram positive bacilli. They appear as small, opaque, enamel-white circular colonies. Cells can measure from 0.5 to 0.8μm by 1.5μm. Transmission electron micrograph of *P. acnes* showed the outer cell wall in lined with cytoplasmic membrane. In the centre is a nucleoid surrounded by ribosomes. Mesosomes are also present (Figure 2).

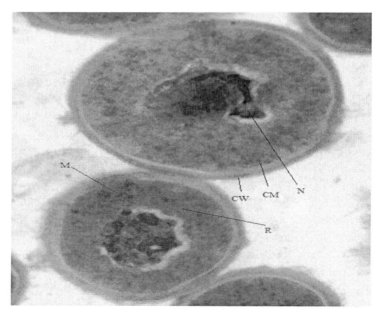

Figure 2. Transmission Electron micrographs of a thin section of *Propionibacterium acnes*. Labelled structures: cell wall (CW), cytoplasmic membrane (CM), nucleoid (N), ribosomes (R) and mesosomes (M).

Cutaneous *Propionibacteria* secrete nucleases, nuraminidases and hyaluronidases, acid phosphatases lecithinases and other lipases. It was suggested that hyaluronidase can split extracellular substance of cell wall of sebaceous ducts and thus increase the permeability of epithelial follicles. Nuraminidase can damage the cell and tissue membranes, affecting the sialic acid residues on surface of the cells. Under the action of proteases of *P. acnes*, which also possesses keratinolytic activity, small chemotactic peptides are produced that may have a role in the onset of inflammation (Vorobjeva, 1999).

6. Pathogenesis of Propionibacterium Acnes

The pathogenesis of acne vulgaris is multifactorial, including increased sebum production, comedogenesis, *P. acnes* proliferation, and inflammation (James, 2003). An increased secretion of sebum is accompanied by thickening of epidermis at the outlet to the pilosebaceous follicles. This creates an obstruction to flow, and a comedo develops. Colonization of the follicle with *P. acnes* and the host inflammatory response to this plays a pivotal role in the development of the typical inflammatory papulopustular lesion (Shaw and Kennedy, 2007). The newest data concerning acne pathophysiology demonstrate that the relationships between the development of *P. acnes*, inflammation, and hyperkeratinization are more complex than previously recognized. Theories regarding the sequence of events in acne development have evolved in recent years. Firstly, it is known that *P. acnes* contribute to inflammation through activation of the innate immune system, including complement and toll-like receptors, and that peroxisome proliferator-activated receptors partially regulate the production of sebum. Secondly, androgens are known to influence follicular corneocytes—that is, androgens do not just mediate acne through sebaceous gland activity, they also have an impact on keratinization. Thirdly, oxidized lipids in sebum can stimulate inflammatory mediators, and it is clear that inflammatory proteins can mediate acne. These mediators include certain matrix metalloproteinases, which are present in sebum; it has been shown that the production of these matrix metalloproteinases decreases after the resolution of acne lesions with treatment. Fourth, and finally, it also has been shown that the sebaceous gland is part of a neuroendocrine organ; it is not yet known how sebaceous gland activity might be mediated using the neuroendocrine inflammatory apparatus, but this represents an area for potential research in the future (Friedlander et al., 2010).

7. Immunology of Acne

Propionibacterium acnes is the predominant organism living on sebaceous region of skin. It lives from metabolising the triglyceride fraction of sebum and is trigger for inflammatory acne. There is no suitable animal model for acne (Webster and Kim, 2008). *P. acnes* act as immunostimulator which produce a variety of enzymes and biologically active molecules like lipases, proteases, hyaluronidases and chemotactic factors involved in development of inflammatory acne.

The main components of the pilosebaceous unit on the skin, such as keratinocytes and sebocytes, can be activated by *P. acnes*, leading to the production of pro-inflammatory cytokines (Leeming et al., 1985). *P. acnes* induce monocytes to secrete pro-inflammatory cytokines like interleukins (IL-8, IL-1β) and tumor necrosis factor (TNF)-α (Kim, 2005) and thus play an important role in pathogenesis of inflammatory acne (Figure 3).

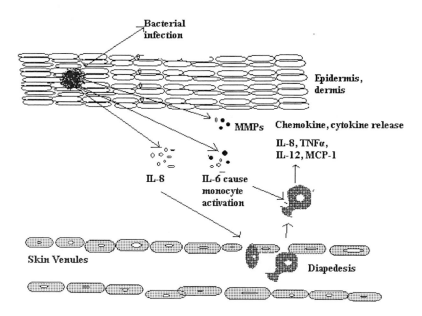

Figure 3. Inflammation of skin in response to the bacterial infection.

P. acnes produce both high and low molecular weight chemotactic factors, one of which is lipase which attract human neutrophils. Once neutrophils arrive, enzymatic digestion of follicular wall occurs by neutrophil lysosomal hydrolytic enzymes. *P. acnes* itself also elaborates proteases and other degradative enzymes, which play some part in comedonal rupture and thus cause inflammation. They induce inflammatory response by activating innate immune cells, such as monocytes/macrophages to secrete proinflammatory cytokines, including IL-8, matrix metalloproteins (MMP), and tumor necrosis factor (TNF) (Fig 4) through TLR2-dependent mechanism (Webster and Kim, 2008).

The innate immune cells i.e. macrophages express pattern recognition receptors (PRRs), such as human TLRs, which are transmembrane proteins capable of mediating responses to pathogen-associated molecular patterns (PAMPs). When TLRs are activated by exposure to microbial ligands, various factors are activated which ultimately activate nuclear factor kappa B (NF-kB) that initiates tumor necrosis factor (TNF α), interleukin and matrix metalloproteins (MMP) (Webster and Kim, 2008). The TLR2-dependent production of IL-8 may be important in the pathogenesis of acne, as it is a known neutrophil chemo attractant, which contribute to the formation of inflammatory lesion. Matrix metalloproteins (MMP) play a role in inducing inflammation and scar formation in acne (Webster and Kim, 2008).

8. Conventional Drugs Available for Treating Acne

Since there is a correlation between the reduction in *P. acnes* number and clinical improvement in patients adequately treated with antimicrobial agents and/or antibiotic therapy, which reduces the population of *P. acnes*, has been a mainstay of treatment for acnes over the past 25 years.

The structured approach for treating acne is as follows:

- *For mild acne*: Topical treatment indicated like use of a comedolytic (retinoid, benzoyl peroxide OR azelaic acid).
- *Possible side-effects*: Benzoyl peroxide and retinoid cause dryness, redness and irritation of skin. Benzoyl peroxide also bleach clothes and hair whereas, azelaic acid leads to hypopigmentation.

- *For moderate acne*: Oral plus topical treatment indicated. Oral antibiotic like tetracycline if over 12 years of age, erythromycin, if younger.
- *Possible side-effects*: Tetracyclines can be associated with photosensitivity, and patients should be cautious in terms of sun exposure. Erythromycin cause frequent gastrointestinal disorders.
- *For severe acne*: Oral plus topical treatment with Dianette or Isotretinoin. A surgery may be recommended in extreme conditions.
- *Possible side effects*: Dianette is associated with an increased risk of venous thromboembolism. Skin and mucous membrane dryness occur in almost all who are treated with Isotretinoin (Shaw and Kennedy, 2007).

Antibiotics have been implemented in the treatment of *P. acnes* due to their bacteriostatic nature, which reduces the pathogen numbers, lipase activity and chemotactic factors produced by the infection of the pathogen. Commonly used antibacterial- clindamycin, erythromycin and tetracycline are all from biological sources, more specifically bacteria. Erythromycin (Scaglione and Rossoni, 1998), retinoids and tretinoin (Wolf, 2002) are used as anti-inflammatory drugs for acne. Clindamycin originates from *Streptomyces lincolnensis*, Erythromycin - *Streptomyces erythreus;* and Tetracycline - *Streptomyces species*. The crisis of newly emerging diseases and the resistance of many pathogens to currently used drugs, coupled with the adverse side-effects of many of these drugs have necessitated the continuous search for new drugs that are potent and efficacious with minimal or no adverse side-effects (Amoo, 2009). However, *P. acnes* strains with clinically significant antibiotic resistance are identified from acne patients with long antibiotic treatments (Ross et al., 1997) to both erythromycin and clindamycin due to their long-term viability as topical anti-acne therapies. Only through judicious use of combination topical therapies (e.g., topical retinoid, benzoyl peroxide or azelaic acid plus clindamycin or erythromycin) can both clindamycin's and erythromycin's widespread utility be preserved in this disorder (Guay, 2007). The reported resistant strain of *P. acne* is P 37 which is erythromycin resistant (Ross et al., 1997). More recently it has been demonstrated that biofilm formation by *P. acnes* increases resistance against antimicrobial agents (Coenye et al., 2007). These problems may be the roots of clinical failure to treat the acne.

The plant kingdom is known to contain many novel biologically active compounds, many of which could potentially have a higher medicinal value when compared to some of the current medications. So there arises a need for search of new effective bioactive compounds to overcome this. A well-known plant extract studied for acne treatment, Tea tree oil or Melaleuca oil, originating from the Australian medicinal plant *Melaleuca alternifolia*, has been used in a clinical trial study to determine its effectiveness against acne (Carson et al., 2006). A crude drug extract called Kushen that is made from the fried roots of *Sophora flavescens* (Leguminosae) contained Prenylflavanone derivatives which were shown to have antibacterial activity against *P. acne* (Kuroyanagi et al., 1995). During previous studies *Hemidesmus indicus*, *Eclipta alba*, *Cucubito pepo*, *Euphorbia hirta* showed minimum inhibitory concentration (MIC) of 0.051mg/ml, 0.665mg/ml, 1.25mg/ml, 1.55mg/ml respectively (Kumar et al., 2007). Rhinacanthins-rich *Rhinacanthus nasutus* extract exhibited potent bacterioststic activity against *P. acnes* with MIC of 8-16µg/ml (Puttarak et al., 2010). The antibacterial activity of pomegranate rind extract containing 13% w/w ellagic acid exibited a bacteriostatic activity against *P. acnes* with a MIC of 15.6µg/ml (Panichayupakaranant et al., 2010). Methanolic extracts of *Rosa damascene*, *Eucommia ulmoides* and *Ilex paraguariensis* were found to inhibit the growth of *P. acnes* with MICs of 2, 0.5 and 1 mg/ml (Tsai et al., 2010). South Africa has remarkable bio diversity and a rich, extant herbal medicine tradition with origins that probably reach back to Paleolithic times. It is estimated that there are at least 200 000 indigenous healers in South Africa. Medicinal plants are widely used in traditional therapeutics, and it is likely that at least 2500 species of plant are commonly used as medicines. A South African pharmaceutical company, Noristan Ltd, investigated South African medicinal plants over a period of almost 20 years. Noristan found that 80% of the local medicinal plants that they had tested exhibited pharmacological activity (Normann and Snyman, 1996). There are many South African plants which are used in herbal cosmetics. Rooibos (*Aspalathus linearis*) is rich in flavanoids, polyphenols, phenolic acids, oligosaccharides and polysaccharides (Dos et al., 2005). Rooibos proved to exhibit anti-inflammatory and anti-microbial properties in cosmetic applications. *Artemisia herba-alba* is also popular for skin ailments. A poultice of leaf is applied to any glandular or skin inflammation (Dweck, 1995). The leaves and roots of *Aloe ferox* are applied topically, sometimes mixed with animal fat, or taken internally to treat conditions such as eczema, dermatitis and acne (Van Wyk et al., 1997). Therefore, there is a wide scope to obtain new drugs from plants that can have potential as antibacterial, anti-inflammatory and anti-oxidant agents.

NOTE: The figures without reference are author's own copy.

References

Amoo, S.O., 2009. Micropropagation and medicinal properties of Barleria greenii and Huernia hystrix. *Biological and Conservation Sciences Theses* 413-653.

Burlando, B., Verotta, L, Comara, L., Bottini-Massa, E., 2010. Herbal Principles in Cosmetics: *Properties and Mechanisms of Action CRC Press*, USA, pp. xxi.

Carson, C.F., Hammer, K.A., Riley, T.V., 2006. *Melaleuca alternifolia* (Tea Tree) Oil: a Review of Antimicrobial and Other Medicinal Properties. *Clinical microbiology reviews* 19, 50-62.

Coenye, T., Peeters, E., Nelis, H.J., 2007. Biofilm formation by *Propionibacterium acnes* is associated with increased resistance to antimicrobial agents and increased production of putative virulence factors. *Research in microbiology* 158, 386-392.

Dos, A., Ayhan, Z., Sumnu, G., 2005. Effects of different factors on sensory attributes, overall acceptance and preference of rooibos (*Aspalathus linearis*) tea. *Journal of Sensory Studies* 20(3), 228–242.

Dweck, A.C., 1995. *Cosmetics and toiletries advanced technology conference.* In: Botanicals - Research of Actives.

Friedlander, S.F., Eichenfield, L.F., Fowler Jr, J.F., Fried, R.G., Levy, M.L., Webster, G.F., 2010. *Acne Epidemiology and Pathophysiology.* Seminars in cutaneous medicine and surgery 29, 2-4.

Gebelein, C.G., 1997. Colin, H., Wheatley (Eds.), Chemistry and Our Life. Graphic World Publishing Services, United States of America, pp. 435–456.

Guay D.R., 2007. Topical clindamycin in the management of acne vulgaris. *Expert Opinion Pharmacotherapy* 8(15), 2625-64.

Hartshorne, S.T., 2003. Dermatological disorders in Johannesburg, South Africa. *Clinical and experimental dermatology* 28, 661-665.

Hoffmann, F.W., Manning, M., 2002. *Herbal medicine and botanical medical fads*. The Haworth Press, Binghamton.

James J, L., 2003. A review of the use of combination therapies for the treatment of acne vulgaris. *Journal of the American Academy of Dermatology* 49, S200-S210.

Kim J. , 2005. Review of the Innate Immune Response in Acne vulgaris: Activation of Toll-Like Receptor 2 in Acne Triggers Inflammatory Cytokine Responses. *Dermatology* 211(3), 193-8.

Kumar, G, S., Jayaveera, K .N ., Kumar, C .K., Sanjay, U. P., Swamy, B .M., Kumar, D, V. , 2007. Antimicrobial effects of Indian medicinal plants against acne-inducing bacteria. *Tropical Journal of Pharmaceutical Research* 6(2), 717-723.

Kuroyanagi, M., Arakawa, T., Hirayama, Y., Hayashi, T., 1995. - Antibacterial and Antiandrogen Flavonoids from Sophora flavescens. - *Journal of Natural Products* 62(12), - 1595.

Leeming, J.P., Holland, K.T., Cunliffe, W.J., 1985. The pathological and ecological significance of microorganisms colonising acne vulgaris comedones. *Journal of medical microbiology* 20, 11-16.

Mantle, D., Gok M.A., Lennard, T.W., 2001. - Adverse and beneficial effects of plant extracts on skin and skin disorders. - Adverse drug reactions and toxicological reviews 20(2), 89-103.

Normann, H., Snyman, I., 1996. Relationship between the sources of traditional and western medicine. *Indigenous knowledge and its uses in southern Africa*, HSRC Publishers, Pretoria, pp. 45.

Panichayupakaranant, P., Tewtrakul, S., Yuenyongsawad, S. , 2010. Antibacterial, anti-inflammatory and anti-allergic activities of standardised pomegranate rind extract. *Food Chemistry* 123, 400-403.

Puttarak, P., Charoonratana, T., Panichayupakaranant, P., 2010. Antimicrobial activity and stability of rhinacanthins-rich Rhinacanthus nasutus extract. *Phytomedicine* 17, 323-327.

Ross, J.I., Eady, E.A., Cove, J.H., Jones, C.E., Ratyal, A.H., Miller, Y.W., Vyakrnam, S., Cunliffe, W.J. , 1997. Clinical resistance to erythromycin and clindamycin in cutaneous propionibacteria isolated from acne patients is associated with mutations in 23S rRNA. *Antimicrobial Agents and Chemotherapy* 41, 1162-1165.

Scaglione, F.,Rossoni, G. , 1998. Comparative anti-inflammatory effects of roxithromycin, azithromycin and clarithromycin. *Journal of Antimicrobial Chemotherapy* 41, 47-50.

Shaw, L., Kennedy, C. , 2007. The treatment of acne. *Paediatrics and Child Health* 17, 385-389.

Spiewak, R., 2000. Occupational skin diseases among formers. *Occupational and Para-Occupational Diseases in Agriculture*. Zagorski, J. (Ed.).

Spinella, M., 2005. Introduction. *Concise handbook of psychoactive herbs*. The Haworth Herbal Press, Binghamton, pp. 1.

Truter, I., 2009. *Acne vulgaris*. SA Pharmaceutical Journal

Tsai, T., Tsai, T., Wu, W., Tseng, J.T., Tsai, P. , 2010. In vitro antimicrobial and anti-inflammatory effects of herbs against *Propionibacterium acnes*. *Food Chemistry* 119, 964-968.

Van Wyk, B.E., Oudtshoorn, B., Gericke, N., 1997. *Medicinal plants of South Africa*. Briza Publication, Pretoria.

Vorobjeva, L.I., 1999. The genus *Propionibacteria*. Propionibacteria, Kluwer Academic Publishers, Netherlands, pp. 34,35.

Webster, G.F., Kim, J., 2008. The Immunology Of Acne. In: Anthony Gaspari, Stephen K. Tyring. (Eds.), *Clinical and Basic Immunodermatology*, Springer, London, pp. 217-222.

Williams, D. F., Schmitt, W. H., 1996. Skin care Products. Chemistry and technology of the cosmetics and toiletries industry, *Blackie Academic and Proffessional*, London.

Wolf, J., 2002. Potential anti-inflammatory effects of topical retinoids and retinoid analogues. *Advances in Therapy* 19, 109-118.

Yahya, H., 2009. Acne vulgaris in Nigerian adolescents ? prevalence, severity, beliefs, perceptions, and practices. *International journal of dermatology* 48, 498-505.

In: Acne
Editor: Mohamed L. Elsaie

ISBN: 978-1-62618-358-2
© 2013 Nova Science Publishers, Inc.

Chapter II

Acne: Pathogenesis, Therapy and Social Effects

Gabriella Fabbrocini, Sara Cacciapuoti, Dario Bianca and Giuseppe Monfrecola

Section of Dermatology- Department of Medicine
and Surgery University of Naples Federico II - Naples Italy

Abstract

Acne vulgaris is a common skin condition with substantial cutaneous and psychologic disease burden. The emotional impact of acne is comparable to that experienced by patients with systemic diseases, like diabetes and epilepsy. Its pathophysiology is multifactorial and complex, including obstruction of the pilosebaceous unit due to increased sebum production, abnormal keratinization, proliferation of Propionibacterium acnes and inflammation. Topical agents (retinoids, benzoyl peroxide and antibacterials) are the most commonly used therapy for acne. Newer topical therapy, such as photodynamic therapy, has been proposed to increase efficacy when conventional therapies are ineffective. This chapter discusses the etiology, pathogenesis, treatment and psychological impact of acne vulgaris.

Introduction

Acne vulgaris is a disease of the pilosebaceous units, clinically characterized by seborrhea, comedones, papules, pustules, nodules and, in some cases, scarring. Acne is a very common disease affecting all ages and ethnic groups. clinical features characterising different acne clinical types.

Table 1. Different acne clinical types

Clinical types	Clinical Features	Subjects more frequently affected	Evolution
Acne neonatorum	closed comedones on the forehead, nose, and cheeks	Newborns	Spontaneous resolution within four months without scarring
Infantile acne	Comedones/ inflammatory papulopustules to cysts.	Children at 3 to 6 months	This patients may develop severe acne as teenagers.
Acne vulgaris	Microcomedones Closed comedones (whiteheads) Open comedones (blackheads) Papules Pustules Nodules Cysts	Teenagers, but also adult	Unpredictable with the tendency to complete or incomplete remissions in adult
Adult acne	Papules Pustules Nodules Cysts Seborrea	It can be already present or appear de novo in adulthood	Unpredictable
Acne conglobata	Cystic abscesses Confluent follicular and perifollicular inflammations Intercommunicating cysts	Patients from 15 to 25 years of age with an antecedent history in most cases of acne vulgaris of varying degrees of severity.	Serious and disfiguring scars

Clinical types	Clinical Features	Subjects more frequently affected	Evolution
Acne inversa	Recurrent draining sinuses and abscesses in skin folds that carry terminal hairs and apocrine glands	Male and female from the puberty	Healing occurs with substantial scarring
Acne fulminans	ulcerative nodules associated with systemic complications: hematologic manifestations arthritis musculoskeletal symptoms	Caucasian adolescent males	Potentially fatal with systemic involvement
Acne cosmetica and iatrogenic acne	papules and pustules monomorphous in their appearance often associated with systemic signs of drug toxicity	Female using cosmetic containing comedogenic substances or patients assuming drugs that can cause or exacerbate acne	Remission after discontinuing drug
Acne excoriée	excoriated areas with inflammation and superficial crusting	females with psychological problems	Frequent scarring sequels caused by picking

It affects 95% and 83% of 16 year old boys and girls respectively, but it is clearly no longer a problem confined to teenagers. In fact, although acne is commonly considered a problem that occurs in adolescence, an increasing number of patients over 25 years of age are consulting for this condition, and most of these are women. The prevalence of adult acne is 3% in men and between 11% and 12% in women with a significant decline from 45 years of age. Moreover, at 40 years of age 1% of men and 5% of women present acne lesions [1, 2]. Acne may cause psychological distress that is associated with suicidal ideation, mental health problems, and affective isolation [3]. Acne is a polymorphic disease with a wide spectrum of severity.

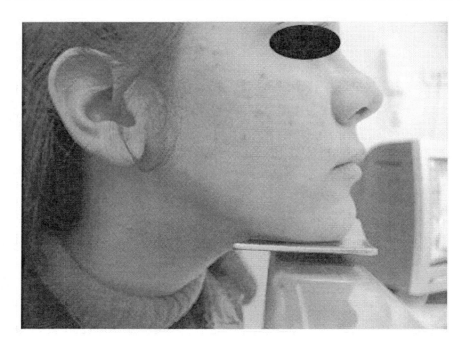

Figure 1. Comedonal acne.

The individual lesions of acne vulgaris are classified into three types: non-inflamed lesions, inflamed lesions and scars. In the first pattern there is increased sebum production on the face, chest, back and shoulders with an increase in pores, blackheads or open comedones (Figure 1). In the second clinical pattern there are papules, pustules, nodules and cysts and any combination of these (Figure 2).

Most patients have a mixture of non-inflamed and inflamed lesions (Figure 3). In some patients, the severe inflammatory lesions result in permanent, disfiguring scars (Figure 4). Acne vulgaris is only one of numerous different and less frequent clinical type of acne. In Table 1 we summarize Although not life-threatening and not a major player in clinical and laboratory research, acne markedly influences quality of life and constitutes a socioeconomic problem.

The worldwide costs for systemic and topical acne treatment were calculated to represent 12.6% of the overall costs for the treatment of skin diseases.

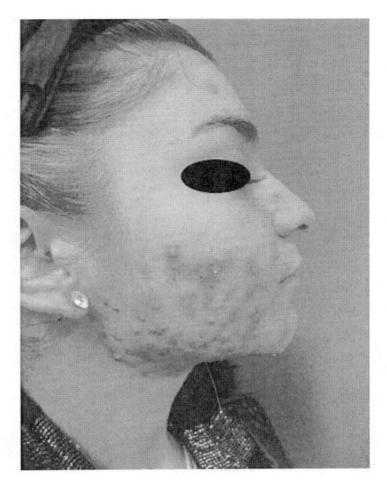

Figure 2. Presence of inflammatory lesions as papules pustules and nodules.

Pathogenesis

Acne is a chronic inflammatory, exclusively human disease of the pilosebaceous unit, mostly affecting the sebaceous gland follicles. The aetiology of acne is not yet fully clarified but it is widely accepted that its pathogenesis is multifactorial, an interplay between a number of factors including:

- hyperkeratinisation with occlusion of the follicular unit
- colonisation by Propionobacterium acnes
- sebum hypersecretion
- inflammation

Hyperkeratinization results in the formation of the primary lesion of acne, the microcomedo. The second key factor involved in acne pathogenesis is the excess sebum production from sebaceous gland. Patients with acne produce more sebum than those without acne and one of the components of sebum, triglycerides, may play a role in acne pathogenesis. In fact triglycerides are broken down into free fatty acids by P. Acnes, promoting further bacterial clumping and colonization of P.Acnes itself, triggering inflammation. P. Acnes is another key element classically involved in acne pathogenesis. P. Acnes is a Gram-positive, anaerobic and microaerobic bacterium found in the sebaceous follicle.

However, recently the role of this bacteria has been reconsidered in light of the fourth, and most important, pathogenetic factor: the inflammation. In fact, recent evidences demonstrate that *P. Acnes* could acts in acne pathogenesis not as pathogen by itself, but by triggering inflammation indirectly. Several immunological targets are involved in this process, such as Toll-like receptors (TLRs). TLRs, localized predominantly in the membrane of immune cells, are the major sensors of the recognition arm of the innate immune system.

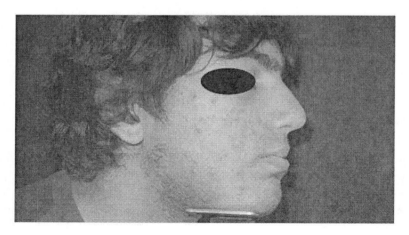

Figure 3. Combination of inflammatory and non-inflammatory lesions.

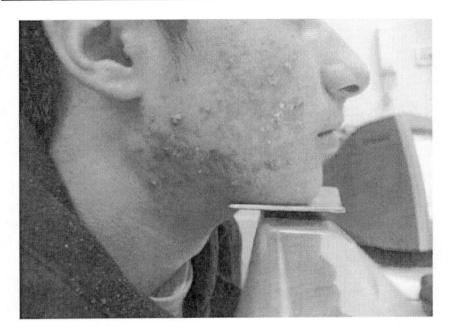

Figure 4. Severe inflammatory lesions with initial scars.

The engagement of these receptors by *P. Acnes* prompts the activation of the networks of innate immunity signalling pathways leading to the activation of nuclear transcription factors responsible for the transcription of inflammatory/immune response-associated genes and the production of a great number of different cytokines, such as TNF-α, IL-1β e IL-8. Moreover, it has been found that *P. acnes* significantly induced human beta-defensin-2 (hBD2) and interleukin-8 (IL-8) mRNA expression. *P. acnes*-induced increase in hBD2 and IL-8 gene expression could be inhibited by anti-TLR2 and anti-TLR4 neutralizing antibodies, suggesting that *P. acnes*-induced secretion of soluble factors in keratinocytes are both TLR2 and TLR4 dependent [4, 5]. Even hyperkeratinisation and hyperseborrea seems to act triggering pro-inflammatory mediator production. In 2003 Jeremy et al. [6] provided newer evidence for the involvement of inflammatory events in the very earliest stages of acne lesion development: inflammatory events occur prior to and act as possible causal factors in the hyperproliferative changes observed in acne lesions, as opposed to secondary consequential events. These data confirm the hypothesis that acne could be an inflammatory disease *ab initio* and that inflammation could be considered the central event in acne pathogenesis (Figure).

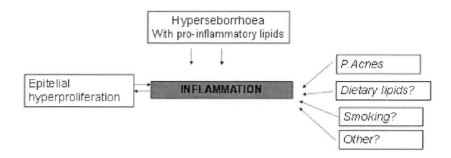

These data suggest that inflammation comes before macroscopically inflamed acne lesion [7] and could explain the basis of ALA-PDT effects on micro- e macrocomedones and could explain the efficacy of some therapeutical approach based on antinflammatory effects even on non-inflammatory lesion (see the case of Photodynamic therapy effects on macro and microcomedones) [8]. More controversial is the role of other factors in which involvement in acne pathogenesis is less clear:

Diet: The current status of the relationship of diet and acne is not clear and under debate. The American Academy of Dermatology published recommendations [9] in 2007 suggesting that there is insufficient evidence to link the consumption of certain food to acne. However, recent studies have suggested a rather close relationship between diet and acne [10, 11]. It's has been hypnotized that the typical Western diet that is a high-glycemic diet could often cause insulin resistance and it could potentiate a change in sebum production and therefore inflammation and acne. With hyperinsulinaemia, there may be an increase in androgen production, resulting in a stimulation of sebaceous glands. It may be that in a small subset of obese acne patients, hyperinsulinaemia may stimulate endogenous androgen production resulting in development or worsening of acne. For this cohort of acne patients, a weight loss diet may be indicated. However, more research is needed to determine whether a low-glycemic diet could effectively mediate acne or possibly even prevent it [12, 13]. *Ultraviolet radiation*: Although an understanding of the photobiology of the skin has been extensively advanced recently, the effect of ultraviolet (UV) radiation on sebaceous glands is not well known. With respect to UV light, it has been reported that in vivo UVB radiation induced hyperplasia of sebaceous glands of hairless mice and hamsters [14, 15]. Clinically, it is said that UV light influences on the pathology of acne development. However, the detailed effects of UV light on sebaceous gland have not been clarified yet. It is known that UV exposure can induce good effects such as vitamin D synthesis, tanning effect, physical wellbeing as well as side effects such as photoallergy, photosensitization, cancer, early aging. In the 1970s up to the 1990s, the frequent short, intermittent and intense sun exposure, due to common holidays in tropical areas have increased sun side effects. Epidemiologic dates suggest that people are often misinformed about sun exposure danger. In Sweden many people use sunbeds to treat certain skin diseases such as acne and seborrhea [16]. Essentially the effects of UV radiation on acne are complex and can be summarized as follow: hyperkeratosis, stimulation of sebaceous secretion, inflammation (all negative for acne evolution), Immunomodulation and hyperpigmentation (that can justify the frequent temporary benefits that acne patients perceive during summer) [17].

Therapy

Of course it is impossible to expound acne therapy without analyzing the main clinical features of the disease. Lesions that characterize acne vulgaris are comedones, papules, pustules and nodules. The elementary lesions of acne are the comedone, which are classically distinguished in whitehead (closed comedone) and blackhead (open comedone). Closed comedones are the forerunner of inflammatory lesions as papules and pustules. Acne vulgaris is usually classified into four clinical patterns:

- comedonal,
- mild to moderate papulopustular acne,
- severe papulopustular acne with or without small nodules,
- severe nodular acne or conglobate acne.

Comedones are quite the only expression of comedonal acne, while inflammatory lesions are less represented. Of course comedones can be observed also in severe inflammatory forms of acne, but in mild and moderate acne inflammatory lesions are predominant, in particular papules and pustules, more diffused in severe acne. Inflammatory nodules are typical of nodular acne; they are deep, infiltrate lesions that can even be confluent in conglobate acne. Scars are another important sign of severe nodular acne. Most frequent localizations of lesions are face and upper trunk corresponding to a greater presence of sebaceous glands.

Therapy Guidelines

In the table below, we briefly describe the European Guidelines for the treatment of acne vulgaris.

Table 2.

	First line treatment	Second line treatment	Third line treatment	Hormonal alternatives for women
Comedonal acne	Topical retinoids, adapalen is preferred to tretinoin	Benzoyl peroxide (BPO) or azelaic acid	/	Not recommended
Mild to moderate papulopustular acne	BPO + adapalene (f.c.)[1] or BPO + clindamycin (f.c.)	BPO or azelaic acid or systemic antibiotic + adapalene	Isotretinoin or tretinoin + topical erythromycin (f.c.); or systemic antibiotics + BPO; or systemic antibiotics + azelaic acid; systemic antibiotics + adapalene + BPO (f.c.)	Not recommended
Severe papulopustular acne and mild nodular acne	Systemic isotretinoin	Systemic antibiotics + adapalene; or systemic antibiotics + azelaic acid; or systemic antibiotics + BPO + adapalene (f.c.)	Systemic antibiotics + BPO	Hormonal antiandrogens + topical treatment or systemic antibiotics (topical treatment is preferred)
Severe nodular acne and conglobate acne	Systemic Isotretinoin	Systemic antibiotics + azelaic acid	Systemic antibiotics + BPO; or systemic antibiotics + adapalene; or systemic antibiotics + BPO + adapalene (f.c)	Hormonal antiandrogens + systemic antibiotics (consider as third line treatment)

1. fixed combination.

Topical Therapies

Retinoids

Chemistry. *Tretinoin* (retinoic acid or trans-retinoic acid) is the acid form of vitamin A which is physiologically in the alcoholic form. *Isotretinoin* (13-cis-retinoic acid) is an isomer of tretinoin. *Adapalene* is derived from nafhthoic acid but its chemical structure is similar to retinoic acid. Thanks to that it can perform the same molecular actions.

Mechanism of action. These drugs bind two kind of receptors: RAR (retinoic acid receptor) and RXR (retinoic X receptor). Of each receptor three sub-types are currently known (α, β, γ). While tretinoin binds only RAR receptors, adapalene has shown high affinity for RAR-β and RAR-γ, and low affinity for RAR-α and RXR receptors. Currently many effects of retinoids have already been demonstrated. First of all they reduce inflammation. They reduce lipoxygenase activity and leukotriene production. In particular adapalene has shown the greatest activity compared to the other retinoids [18]. Retinoids action also results in lower levels of oxygen free radicals produced by polimorfonucleate neutrophil (PMN); while adapalene even inhibits PMN chemotaxis. At high concentrations of retinoids it is also demonstrated that TLR-2 are less expressed by monocytes. It is important to note, of course, the effects of retinoids on sebocytes. These drugs in fact are able to stop cell differentiation and cell cycle progression, and to induce apoptosis. These effects seem to be mediated not only by the interaction with RAR or RXR but also by the inhibition of other pathways in particular those dependent by FGFR-2 [19, 20]. This pathway seems to be influenced also by other anti-acne agents such as antibiotics and BPO [21].

Clinical indications in acne treatment. Retinoids are the first choice alone in the treatment of comedonal acne. They have shown better outcomes against placebo and against azelaic acid [22-24]. In comparison with BPO retinoids they have shown comparable-to-superior efficacy [25, 26]. Among retinoids, adapalene is preferred for its superior tolerability. In papulopustolar acne topical adapalene is used in combination with BPO and this kind of combination therapy has shown better outcomes than therapy based on adapalene or BPO alone; adapalene + BPO has shown similar results to clindamycin and BPO [23, 27, 28].

As seen before in severe papulopustular and nodular acne topical retinoids are a second line treatment in association with oral antibiotics. Adverse effect of topical retinoids consist mainly in an irritant contact dermatitis. Some authors discuss about the possibility of systemic adverse events related to retinoids topical use.

A review of the literature has recently concluded that systemic adverse effects during topical therapy with retinoids are rare [29]. However they remain an excellent instrument for physicians in acne treatment.

Antibiotics

Our discussion will focus on tetracycline, clindamycin, erythromycin and nadifloxacin, a new emerging antibiotic for acne treatment. With regards to their mechanism of action antibiotics are used in acne therapy for two reasons. Evidently they have an antibacterial activity, inhibiting P. acnes growth by several molecular mechanisms different from molecule to molecule. The second reason is their demonstrated anti-inflammatory activity. Antibiotics are in fact able to reduce chemotaxis and oxygen free radicals produced by PMN and other inflammatory cells, in this way skin inflammatory infiltrate is reduced with consequential reduced skin damage [30, 31]. Tetracycline, once inside bacterial cells, bind 30S sub-unit of bacterial ribosomes managing to prevent protein synthesis by bacteria. Erythromycin and clindamycin instead inhibits production of proteins binding 50S sub-unit of ribosomes on the same site. Nadifloxacine as the other chinolones inhibits bacterial topoisomerase II and IV.

Clinical indications in acne treatment. In comedonal acne all topical antibiotics have shown better activity against placebo [32-35]. However they have lower efficacy in comparison with BPO [36-39]. In mild papulo-pustular acne combination therapy of BPO and clindamycin has shown better efficacy in comparison with BPO alone and adapalene alone. BPO + clindamycin and BPO + adapalene have shown the same efficacy [28]. Nadifloxacine and erythromycin can be a second line alternative to clindamycin [40]. Topical antibiotics should not be used in mono-therapy in order to avoid P. acnes antibiotics resistance.

Also switching from a topical antibiotic to another is not recommended and in case of low efficacy of the topical treatment a systemic antibiotic should be associated. Systemic therapy with an antibiotic is also associated with a lower frequency of adverse events. Some studies have in fact demonstrated that skin xerosis and irritant dermatitis related to topical agents are more likely to induce discontinuation of treatment in comparison with adverse events (mainly gastrointestinal) related to systemic therapy [41, 42].

Benzoyl Peroxide

Chemistry and effects: BPO represents one of the most effective topical agents in the treatment of acne. Once in the epidermis and derma it is metabolized in benzoic acid. Its real effects are not well known yet. Anyway it surely has an antimicrobial activity toward P. acnes. Clinical indications in acne treatment: in comedonal acne BPO is a second line agent, in alternative to retinoids; it has in fact shown lower efficacy when compared to retinoids in this acne form [25, 26, 43]. However, in comparison with topical antibiotics as erythromycin [44], clyndamicyn [37, 38, 45], and tetracycline [39], instead, BPO has shown higher efficacy. Also when compared to azelaic acid BPO gave better outcomes [46, 47]. In mild to moderate papulo-pustular acne BPO is considered the first choice together with adapalene or clindamycin in fixed combination. BPO + adapalene has shown superior efficacy against infiammatory lesions when compared to BPO or adapalene alone [23, 27, 48]. Combination therapy instead of BPO + clindamycin has shown better results when compared to BPO alone or clindamycin alone [36, 49-52]. The two combination therapies have shown comparable efficacy against inflammatory lesions [28]. BPO side effects are mainly represented by an irritant, dose-dependent contact dermatitis, which is more frequent at higher concentrations [53, 54].

Chemical Peels

Chemical peels induce a controlled skin damage with consequent activation of inflammatory cascade. Skin damage results in improvement of cell turnover. Different agents have different depths of penetration, and therefore, chemical peels can be divided into 3 different groups based on the histologic level of necrosis that they cause.

1) Superficial: destruction of the only corneum stratum (Glycolic acid 30-70%, Salicylic acid 15% , TCA 10% , Mandelic acid 30%)

2) Medium: destruction of the epidermis and part or all of the papillary dermis (Glycolic acid 70%, piruvic acid 30%, Azelaic acid 30%, Salicylic acid 33%)
3) Deep: destruction of the epidermis and papillary dermis, extending into the reticular dermis. TCA 30%, Salicilyc acid 50%

Systemic Therapy

Retinoids

Oral isotretinoin is considered the first line agent for severe papulo-pustular acne, for nodular and conglobate acne. In severe papulo-pustular acne it has shown comparable results in comparison with minocycline and topical azelaic acid. Anyway isotretinoin has also shown faster onset of the results [55]. Treatment with insotretinoin has also demonstrated greater efficacy in comparison with the association of tetracycline and topical adapalene [56]. In nodular and conglobate acne, isotretinoin at the dose of 0,5 mg/kg brought to a reduction of nodules and cysts of about 70% [57-59]. According to the latest guidelines for the treatment of acne, isotretinoin should be used as soon as possible in severe inflammatory acne and when nodules and cysts are present in order to avoid clinical scars. The dose should be comprised between 0,3-0,5 mg/kg die in papulo-pustular acne and even ≥ 0.5 mg/kg in nodular and conglobate acne. The treatment should last for at least 6 months. Liver enzymes and lipids should be tested 1 month before the treatment, 1 month after the beginning of the treatment and every 3 months of treatment. This kind of therapy is not recommended in children younger than 12 years old. Laser treatment and peeling must be avoided during the treatment and after 6 months from the stopping. Because of the risks in case of pregnancy, young women should adopt 2 methods of contraception during the treatment, 1 month before the beginning and 1 month after the end of therapy. Physicians must also require a pregnancy test 1 month before and every month after the start of therapy. The main side effects are headache, skin dryness and depression until suicide. The real incidence of this last side effect is controversial and even if the current literature seems to exclude an association between isotretionin and depression the Authors underline that all the most important studies have great limitations [60].

Oral Antibiotics

The most important antibiotics used for the systemic treatment of acne are tetracycline, in particular minocycline, doxycycline and limecycline, and macrolides, in particular erythromycin. Antibiotic therapy is suggested as second line treatment of moderate inflammatory acne which does not respond to topical therapy and in case of patients with severe or nodular acne for whom systemic retinoids are not indicated. Oral antibiotics have shown better results when associated with topical retinoids. In particular the association of topical adapalene + oral doxycycline and the association of topical adapalene + BPO + oral doxycycline have shown better results in comparison with doxycycline alone [61, 62]. Also limecycline gave better outcomes when associated with adapalene [63]. Concerning antibiotics tolerability a review by Smith and Leyden demonstrated a higher incidence of severe side effects with minocycline in comparison with doxycycline. In fact although doxycycline leads to photosensitivity that is not induced by minocycline, we prefer the use of doxycycline because of the easier management of its side effects. Photo-induced skin damage during the treatment with doxycycline in fact can be obviously prevented using sun protection, and esophagitis, another potential side effect of doxycycline, can be prevented with a sufficient water intake together with the pill assumption. In any case the most important problem of antibiotic therapy is surely the risk of antibiotic resistance. This kind of phenomenon is more and more increasing and in some countries it has reached worrying characteristics for erythromycin and clyndamicin (in Spain it seems that the prevalence of resistance to erythromycin and clyndamicin is over 90%) while is less frequent for tetracyclines. Moreover the observation of dangerous infection due to multi-resistant P. acnes (e.g. after surgery) has led to more strict recommendations to the use of antibiotics in acne treatment. In particular topical monotherapy should be avoided and the use of antibacterials as BPO could be a good solution to avoid resistance.

What's New

Photodynamic Therapy

Several studies have shown that ALA-PDT can lead to prolonged improvement in acne [64-66]. In a systematic review with an evidence-based approach to assess the effects of optical treatments for acne vulgaris, original publications of controlled clinical trials were identified through searches in PubMed and the Cochrane Library [67]. The authors concluded that optical treatments possess the potential to improve inflammatory acne on a short-term basis with the most consistent outcomes for PDT [up to 68% improvement, ALA, methyl-aminolevulinic acid (MAL) and red light]. ALA-PDT is a two-step therapeutic technique in which the delivery of photosensitizing drugs is followed by irradiation with visible light. Activated photosensitizers transfer energy to molecular oxygen, generating reactive oxygen species (ROS). The subsequent oxidation of lipids, amino acids and proteins induces cell necrosis and apoptosis. Using the intrinsic cellular haem biosynthetic pathway and principles of photoillumination, topical PDT selectively targets abnormal cells, while preserving the normal surrounding structures. ALA is not a photosensitizer by itself but it is metabolized to photosensitive protoporphyrin IX (PpIX) through the intrinsic cellular haem biosynthetic pathway. Topically applied, 5-ALA and its derivatives take advantage of the intrinsic cellular haem biosynthetic pathway to produce photoactive porphyrins. Using a series of enzymatic reactions between the mitochondria and the cytosol, ALA is ultimately converted to protoporphyrin IX [68]. Pp IX is a photosensitizer that accumulates not only in the epidermal cells but also in the pilosebaceous units. This fluorescent molecule, through its extensive network of alternating double bonds, is essential to the transfer of singlet oxygen species and the formation of free radicals, which result in cellular damage to various organelles, including the mitochondria and endoplasmic reticulum, as well as the plasma membrane [69]. The rationale for the use of PDT in the treatment of acne is based on the knowledge that P. Acnes contain endogenous porphyrins. Additionally, selectivity of ALA-induced porphyrin fluorescence for pilosebaceous units has been shown in animal models [70].

Social Effects

In modern Society the ideal of perfect skin makes appearance the most important factor. Embarrassment and self-consciousness are directly linked to self-image and self-esteem. For these reasons it is known by physicians how acne vulgaris can have significant non-dermatological effect in the specific population affected due to the strong emphasis placed on physical appearance. Psychiatric disorders can develop secondary to acne vulgaris [71-73]. Some studies have found that depression is more prevalent among patients with acne than among control subjects [74-76]. Other uncontrolled studies have found rates of depression higher among those with acne than is the norm [72, 77, 78]. Depression, anxiety, and overall psychiatric morbidity have been found to improve when acne is treated (especially with isotretinoin therapy) [79, 80].

Acne has been implicated in psychiatric and psychological processes more than most other dermatological conditions. Acne patients report greater levels of anxiety and depression than other medical populations, including cancer patients and other dermatology patients [72] such as alopecia areata, atopic dermatitis, and mild-to-moderate psoriasis. The only group, that surpassed acne with incidence of clinical depression and suicidal ideation were in patients with severe psoriasis. Studies have found significant impairment in self-image and self-esteem, impairment in psychological well-being, dissatisfaction with appearance, and inhibition of social interactions in acne patients [79, 81-83].

There are many aspects of this disease that contribute to its non dermatological effects including predominant anatomical distribution of lesions, misperceptions regarding etiology, and social pressures, and ,first of all, adolescent prevalence. Acne is the most frequent visible skin disease in adolescents. In adolescence, the individual usually becomes increasingly autonomous. The relationship with family members changes, peer and romantic relationships become more important, and enduring relationships may begin. Adolescence is known to be a period especially associated with psychological distress. Adolescents are psychologically vulnerable, and they tend to be sensitive to modifications in their bodies and appearance. Girls and boys with acne have lower self-confidence, more feelings of uselessness, fewer feelings of pride, lower self-worth, and lower body satisfaction than those without acne. Adolescents tend also to have bad habits that can even worsen acne. In particular the use of sunbeds to cure acne and skin pathologies is about 35% and it is related to socioeconomical status. In Italy young people are very aware of the risks associated with sunbathing but they preferred to be tanned and sunbathe to be more attractive (75%of the sample) [84]. In a regression model for body mass index and depressive symptoms, acne explains significantly lower self-attitude (for boys) and poor self-worth (for girls). Social relations affect physical and mental health and vice versa. The appearance of the skin is important in social interaction and for self-image. The severe burden of acne is a strong justification for effective acne treatment and psychiatric screening for patients with the condition. It is therefore necessary to detect psychological suffering, depression, anxiety, and (especially) suicidal ideations, as well as other psychiatric diseases in adolescents with acne, and to propose appropriate treatment. Because of the role of acne in depression and suicidal ideations (or their frequency), it is also necessary to effectively treat acne itself. Among the options, isotretinoin is indicated for severe acne, but it has been considered a potential trigger factor for suicide in predisposed subject. A great number of reports on its effects have been published since its introduction into the market. However, a causal relationship has not been established and the link between isotretinoin use and psychiatric events remains controversial. A review including all published material reporting psychiatric side effects following isotretinoin treatment [85]. The authors concluded that a link between isotretinoin and psychopathology was possible but not restricted to depression and that there was a need for placebo-controlled prospective studies to establish a causal link. Acne appears to be an independent risk factor for suicidal ideation, especially in boys. For these reasons adverse events that have been attributed to therapies for acne, including suicidal ideation and depression, may reflect the burden of substantial acne rather than the effect of medications. In fact, clinicians must keep in mind that substantial acne is a major risk factor for depression and suicidal ideation and that it may be necessary to treat patients effectively for both depression and acne. According to some authors in adults acne is associated with even greater psychological effects than in adolescents, especially in female patients. In adulthood acne is associated in particular with physical discomfort and acne [86].

Acne is associated with considerable psychological morbidity. This morbidity is complex and often does not conform to standard psychiatric disease criteria. For these reasons a global approach to acne patients is essential for a correct acne management. In some Clinical Department a dedicated ambulatory is used to follow up acne patients in their clinical and psychological evolution. The division of Clinical Dermatology from the Department of Systematic Pathology of the University of Naples Federico II is one of these structures. Here it has implemented for almost two years now an outpatient office in which global care is provided for patients with acne. At this office the patient's medical history is recorded and notes are taken regarding any treatments she or he has received. Using this global approach Fabbrocini et al. tested Cardiff Disability Index (CADI) [87], a questionnaire that aims to measure the impact of acne on social function and mood, in teenagers and young adults with acne referred to their observation [88]. They found that 57% of the patients enrolled in the study showed that acne causes noticeable discomfort in their lives. However, the data was more evident in females (66%) compared to males (33.5%). The percentage of female patients that experience discomfort was greater in the slight acne stage of the disease demonstrating that, even at a light clinical stage, acne can be a source of distress. In addition, they observed that the length of an acne pathology plays a significant role in the perception of discomfort associated with the disease. In fact, the level of discomfort for patients who have had slight and moderate acne for over 5 years, was quite similar to the level of discomfort of patients who have had severe acne for less than a year. It is important that the dermatologist understands how the young person is experiencing this skin disease, and how acne creates an esthetic uneasiness that can influence their emotional wellbeing.

References

[1] Goulden V et al. Prevalence of facial acne in adults. *J. Am. Acad. Dermatol.* 1999; 41:577-80.
[2] White GM. Recent findings in the epidemiologic evidence, classification, and subtypes of acne vulgaris. *J. Am. Acad. Dermatol.*
[3] Halvorsen JA et al. Suicidal ideation, mental health problems, and social impairment are increased in adolescents with acne: a population-based study. *J. Invest. Dermatol.* 2011 131:363–70.
[4] Jugeau S et al. Induction of toll-like receptors by Propionibacterium acnes. *Br. J. Dermatol.* 2005 Dec; 153(6):1105-13.
[5] Nagy I et al. Distinct strains of Propionibacterium acnes induce selective human beta-defensin-2 and interleukin-8 expression in human keratinocytes through toll-like receptors. *J. Invest. Dermatol.* 2005 May; 124(5):931-8.
[6] Jeremy AH et al. Inflammatory events are involved in acne lesion initiation. *J. Invest. Dermatol.* 2003 Jul; 121(1):20-7.
[7] Takahashi H et al.: Activation of two caspase cascades, caspase 8/3/6 and caspase 9/3/6, during photodynamic therapy using a novel photosensitizer, ATX-S10(Na), in normal human keratinocytes. *Arch. Dermatol. Res.* 2003 Nov; 295(6):242-8. Epub 2003 Sep 11.
[8] Fabbrocini G et al. The effect of aminolevulinic acid photodynamic therapy on microcomedones and macrocomedones. *Dermatology.* 2009; 219(4):322-8. Epub 2009 Oct 23.

[9] Strauss JS et al. American Academy of Dermatology/American Academy of Dermatology Association. Guidelines of care for acne vulgaris management. *J. Am. Acad. Dermatol.* 2007; 56:651-63.
[10] Smith RN et al. A low-glycemic- load diet improves symptoms in acne vulgaris patients: a randomized controlled trial. *Am. J. Clin. Nutr.* 2007; 86:107-15.
[11] Smith RN et al. The effect of a low glycemic load diet on acne vulgaris and the fatty acid composition of skin surface triglycerides. *J. Dermatol. Sci.* 2008; 50:41-52.
[12] Aizawa H et al. Elevated serum insulin-like growth factor-1 (IGF-1) levels in women with postadolescent acne. *J. Dermatol.* 1995; 22:249–52.
[13] Del Prete M et al. Insulin resistance and acne: a new risk factor for men? *Endocrinology* 2012, in press.
[14] Lesnik RH et al. Agents that cause enlargement of sebaceous glands in hairless mice. II. Ultraviolet radiation. *Arch. Dermatol. Res.* 1992;284:106_/8.
[15] Dachs U et al. Effecte des UV-Lichtes auf Hautadnexe am Beispiel des Syrischen Hamsters. *Hautartzt* 1977; 28(Suppl. 2):237_/8.
[16] Boldeman C et al. Sunbed use in relation to phenotype, erythema, sunscreen use and skin diseases. A questionnaire survey among Swedish adolescents. *J. Dermatol.* 1996 Nov; 135(5):712-6.
[17] Yasuchiyo Akitomo et al. Effects of UV irradiation on the sebaceous gland and sebum secretion in hamsters. *J. Dermatol. Sci.* 2003 Apr; 31(2):151-9.
[18] Jones DA The potential immunomodulatory effects of topical retinoids *Dermatology Online Journal* 11 (1): 3.
[19] AM Nelson et al. 13-cis Retinoic Acid Induces Apoptosis and Cell Cycle Arrest in Human SEB-1 Sebocytes *Journal of Investigative Dermatology* (2006) 126, 2178–2189.
[20] Giannini F et al. All-trans, 13-cis and 9-cis retinoic acids induce a fully reversible growth inhibition in HNSCC cell lines: implications for in vivo retinoic acid use. *Int. J. Cancer.* 1997 Jan 17; 70(2):194-200.
[21] Bodo C et al. Anti-Acne Agents Attenuate FGFR2 *Signal Transduction in Acne Journal of Investigative Dermatology* (2009) 129, 1868–1877.
[22] Hughes BR et al. A double-blind evaluation of topical isotretinoin 0.05%, benzoyl peroxide gel 5% and placebo in patients with acne. *Clin. Exp. Dermatol.* 1992; 17; 165-168.

[23] Thiboutot DM et al. Adapalene-benzoyl peroxide, a fixed-dose combination for the treatment of acne vulgaris: results of a multicenter, randomized double-blind, controlled study. *J. Am. Acad. Dermatol.* 2007; 57; 791-799.

[24] Thiboutot D et al. Adapalene gel 0.3% for the treatment of acne vulgaris: a multicenter, randomized, double-blind, controlled, phase III trial. *J. Am. Acad. Dermatol.* 2006; 54; 242-250.

[25] Bucknall JH et al. Comparison of tretinoin solution and benzoyl peroxide lotion in the treatment of acne vulgaris. *Curr. Med. Res. Opin.* 1977; 5; 266-268.

[26] Lyons RE. Comparative effectiveness of benzoyl peroxide and tretinoin in acne vulgaris. *Int. J. Dermatol.* 1978; 17; 246-25.

[27] Gold LS et al. A North American study of adapalene - benzoyl peroxide combination gel in the treatment of acne. *Cutis.* 2009; 84; 110-116.

[28] Zouboulis CC et al. Study of the efficacy, tolerability, and safety of 2 fixed-dose combination gels in the management of acne vulgaris. *Cutis.* 2009; 84; 223-229.

[29] Shapiro S, et al. Use of topical tretinoin and the development of noncutaneous adverse events: evidence from a systematic review of the literature. *J. Am. Acad. Dermatol.* 2011 Dec; 65(6):1194-201. Epub 2011 May 6.

[30] Pinar Y. et al. The effect of benzoyl peroxide and benzoyl peroxide/erythromycin combination on the antioxidative defence system in papulopustular acne. *European Journal of Dermatology.* Volume 12, Number 1, 53-7, January - February 2002, Thérapie.

[31] Anna Bender1 et al. Tetracycline suppresses ATPγS-induced CXCL8 and CXCL1 production by the human dermal microvascular endothelial cell-1 (HMEC-1) cell line and primary human dermalmicrovascular endothelial cells. *Exp. Dermatol.* 2008 September; 17(9): 752–760. doi:10.1111/j.1600-0625.2008.00716.x.

[32] 32 Leyden JJ et al. Two randomized, double-blind, controlled trials of 2219 subjects to compare the combination clindamycin/tretinoin hydrogel with each agent alone and vehicle for the treatment of acne vulgaris. *J. Am. Acad. Dermatol.* 2006; 54; 73-81.

[33] Kuhlman DS et al. A comparison of clindamycin phosphate 1 percent topical lotion and placebo in the treatment of acne vulgaris. *Cutis.* 1986; 38; 203-206.

[34] Mills O, et al. Bacterial resistance and therapeutic outcome following three months of topical acne therapy with 2% erythromycin gelversus its vehicle. *Acta. Derm. Venereol.* 2002; 82; 260-265.
[35] Dobson RL et al. Topical erythromycin solution in acne. Results of a multiclinic trial. *J. Am. Acad. Dermatol.* 1980; 3; 478-482.
[36] Lookingbill DP et al. Treatment of acne with a combination clindamycin/benzoyl peroxide gel compared with clindamycin gel, benzoyl peroxide gel and vehicle gel: combined results of two double-blind investigations. *J. Am. Acad. Dermatol.* 1997; 37; 590-595.
[37] Swinyer LJ et al. A comparative study of benzoyl peroxide and clindamycin phosphate for treating acne vulgaris. *Br. J. Dermatol.* 1988; 119; 615-622.
[38] Tucker SB et al. Comparison of topical clindamycinphosphate, benzoyl peroxide, and a combination of the two for the treatment of acne vulgaris. *Br. J. Dermatol.* 1984; 110; 487-492.
[39] Norris JF et al. A comparison of the effectiveness of topical tetracycline, benzoyl-peroxide gel and oral oxytetracycline in the treatment of acne. *Clin. Exp. Dermatol.* 1991; 16; 31-33.
[40] Jung JY, et al. Clinical and histological evaluation of 1% nadifloxacin cream in the treatment of acne vulgaris in Korean patients. *Int. J. Dermatol.* 2011 Mar; 50(3):350-7.
[41] Gratton D et al. Topical clindamycin versus systemic tetracycline in the treatment of acne. Results of a multiclinic trial. *J. Am. Acad. Dermatol.* 1982; 7; 50-53.
[42] Ozolins M et al. Randomised controlled multiple treatment comparison to provide a cost-effectiveness rationale for the selection of antimicrobial therapy in acne. *Health Technol Assess.* 2005; 9.
[43] Handojo I. The combined use of topical benzoyl peroxide and tretinoin in the treatment of acne vulgaris. *Int. J. Dermatol.* 1979; 18; 489-496.
[44] Burke B et al. Benzoyl peroxide versus topical erythromycin in the treatment of acne vulgaris. *Br. J. Dermatol.* 1983; 108; 199-204.
[45] Tschen EH et al. A combination benzoyl peroxide and clindamycin topical gel compared with benzoyl peroxide, clindamycin phosphate, and vehicle in the treatment of acne vulgaris. *Cutis.* 2001; 67; 165-169.
[46] Stinco G et al. Relationship between sebostatic activity, tolerability and efficacy of three topical drugs to treat mild to moderate acne. *J. Eur. Acad. Dermatol. Venereol.* 2007; 21; 320-325.

[47] Gollnick HP et al. Azelaic acid 15% gel in the treatment of acne vulgaris. Combined results of two double-blind clinical comparative studies. *J. Dtsch. Dermatol. Ges.* 2004; 2; 841-847.

[48] Gollnick HP et al. Adapalenebenzoyl peroxide, a unique fixed-dose combination topical gel for the treatment of acne vulgaris: a transatlantic, randomized, double-blind, controlled study in 1670 patients. *Br. J. Dermatol.* 2009; 161;1180-1189.

[49] Webster G et al. Efficacy and tolerability of a fixed combination of clindamycin phosphate (1.2%) and low concentration benzoyl peroxide (2.5%) aqueous gel in moderate or severe acne subpopulations. *J. Drugs Dermatol.* 2009; 8; 736-743.

[50] Thiboutot D et al. An aqueous gel fixed combination of clindamycin phosphate 1.2% and benzoyl peroxide 2.5% for the once-daily treatment of moderate to severe acne vulgaris: assessment of efficacy and safety in 2813 patients. *J. Am. Acad. Dermatol.* 2008; 59; 792-800.

[51] Ellis CN et al. Therapeutic studies with a new combination benzoyl peroxide/clindamycin topical gel in acne vulgaris. *Cutis.* 2001; 67; 13-20.

[52] Leyden JJ et al. Comparison of the efficacy and safety of a combination topical gel formulation of benzoyl peroxide and clindamycin with benzoyl peroxide, clindamycin and vehicle gel in the treatments of acne vulgaris. *American journal of clinical dermatology.* 2001; 2; 33-39.

[53] Harper JC. Benzoyl peroxide development, pharmacology, formulation and clinical uses in topical fixed-combinations. *J. Drugs Dermatol.* 2010 May; 9(5):482-7.

[54] M, Yentzer BA et al. Benzoyl peroxide: a review of its current use in the treatment of acne vulgaris. *Sagransky Expert Opin. Pharmacother.* 2009 Oct; 10(15):2555-62.

[55] Gollnick HP et al. Comparison of combined azelaic acid cream plus oral minocycline with oral isotretinoin in severe acne. *Eur. J. Dermatol.* 2001; 11; 538-544.

[56] Oprica C et al. Clinical and microbiological comparisons of isotretinoin vs. tetracycline in acne vulgaris. *Acta. Derm. Venereol.* 2007; 87; 246-254.

[57] Strauss JS et al. A randomized trial of the efficacy of a new micronized formulation versus a standard formulation of isotretinoin in patients with severe recalcitrant nodular acne. *J. Am. Acad. Dermatol.* 2001; 45; 187-195.

[58] Al Mishari MA. A study of isotretinoin (Roaccutan) in nodulocystic acne. *Clin. Trials J.* 1986; 23; 1-5.
[59] Mandekou-Lefaki I et al. Low-dose schema of isotretinoin in acne vulgaris. *Int. J. Clin. Pharmacol. Res.* 2003; 23; 41-46.
[60] Marqueling AL et al. Depression and suicidal behavior in acne patients treated with isotretinoin: a systematic review. *Semin. Cutan. Med. Surg.* 2007; 26; 210-220.
[61] Thiboutot DM et al. Combination therapy with adapalene gel 0.1% and doxycycline for severe acne vulgaris: a multicenter, investigator-blind, randomized, controlled study. *Skinmed.* 2005; 4; 138-146.
[62] Gold LS et al. Effective and safe combination therapy for severe acne vulgaris: a randomized, vehicle-controlled, double-blind study of adapalene 0.1%-benzoyl peroxide 2.5% fixed-dose combination gel with doxycycline hyclate 100 mg. *Cutis.* 2010; 85; 94-104.
[63] Cunliffe WJ et al. Is combined oral and topical therapy better than oral therapy alone in patients with moderate to moderately severe acne vulgaris? A comparison of the efficacy and safety of lymecycline plus adapalene gel 0.1%, versus lymecycline plus gel vehicle. *J. Am. Acad. Dermatol.* 2003; 49; S218-226.
[64] Hongcharu W et al. Topical ALA-photodynamic therapy for the treatment of acne vulgaris. *Invest. Dermatol.* 2000 Aug; 115(2):183-92.
[65] Pollock B et al. Topical aminolaevulinic acid-photodynamic therapy for the treatment of acne vulgaris: a study of clinical effectiveness and mechanism of action. *Br. J. Dermatol.* 2004 Sep; 151(3):616-22.
[66] Seok-Beom Hong et al. Topical aminolevulinic acid- photodynamic therapy for the treatment of acne vulgaris. *Photodermatol. Photobiol. Photomed.* 2005; 21: 322-325.
[67] Haedersdal M et al. Evidence-based review of lasers, light sources and photodynamic therapy in the treatment of acne vulgaris. *J. Eur. Acad. Dermatol. Venereol.* 2008 Mar; 22(3):267-78.
[68] Kennedy JC et al. Photodynamic therapy with endogenous protoporphyrin IX—basic principles and present clinical experience. *J. Photochem. Photobiol. B Biol.* 1990; 6: 143–8.
[69] Barr H et al. Clinical aspects of photodynamic therapy. *Sci. Prog.* 2002; 85: 131–50.
[70] Divaris DX et al. Phototoxic damage to sebaceous glands and hair follicles of mice after systemic administration of 5-aminolevulinic acid correlates with localized protoporphyrin IX fluorescence. *Am. J. Pathol.* 1990; 136: 891-897.

[71] Kellett SC et al. The psychological and emotional impact of acne and the effect of treatment with isotretinoin. *Br. J. Dermatol.* 1999; 140:273-82.
[72] Gupta MA et al. Depression and suicidal ideation in dermatology patients with acne, alopecia areata, atopic dermatitis and psoriasis. *Br. J. Dermatol.* 1998; 139:846-50.
[73] Cotterill JA et al. Suicide in dermatological patients. *Br. J. Dermatol.* 1997; 137:246-50.
[74] Yazici K et al. Disease-specific quality of life is associated with anxiety and depression in patients with acne. *J. Eur. Acad. Dermatol. Venereol.* 2004; 18:435-9.
[75] Sayar K et al. The psychometric assessment of acne vulgaris patients. *Dermatol. Psychosom.* 2001; 1:62-5.
[76] Khan MZ et al. Prevalence of mental health problems in acne patients. *J. Ayub. Med. Coll. Abbottabad.* 2001; 13:7-8.
[77] Preston K. Depression and skin diseases. *Med. J. Aust.* 1969; 1(7):326-9.
[78] Polenghi MM et al. Emotions and acne. *Dermatol. Psychosom.* 2002; 3:20-5.
[79] Layton AM. Psychosocial aspects of acne vulgaris. *J. Cutan. Med. Surg.* 1998; 2(Suppl3):19-23.
[80] Newton JN et al. The effectiveness of acne treatment: an assessment by patients of the outcome of therapy. *Br. J. Dermatol.* 1997;137(4):563-7.
[81] Van der Meeren et al. The psychological impact of severe acne. *Cutis* 1985; 36:84-6.
[82] Krowchuk DP et al. The psychosocial effects of acne in adolescents. *Pediatric Dermatol.* 1991; 8:332-8.
[83] Klassen AF et al. Measuring quality of life in people referred for specialist care of acne: Comparing generinc and disease-specific measures. *J. AM. Acad. Dermatol.* 2000; 43:229-33.
[84] Monfrecola G et al. What do young people think about the dangers of sunbathing, skin cancer and sunbeds? A questionnaire survey among Italians. Photoderm, *Photoimmunol and Photomedicine*; 2000; 16 : 15-8.
[85] Kontaxakis VP et al. Isotretinoin and psychopathology: a review. *Ann. Gen. Psychiatry.* 2009 Jan 20; 8:2.
[86] GK Pruthi et al. Physical and psychosocial impact of acne in adult females. *Indian Journal of Dermatology* 2012; 57; 26-29.
[87] Motley RJ et al. Practical use of a disability index in the routine management of acne. *Clin. Exp. Dermatol.* 1992; 17:1-3.
[88] Fabbrocini G et al. Quality of life in acne patient. *European Journal of Acne and Related Diseases* Volume 1, n. 1, 2010.

In: Acne
Editor: Mohamed L. Elsaie

ISBN: 978-1-62618-358-2
© 2013 Nova Science Publishers, Inc.

Chapter III

Selected Thai Medicinal Plant for the Treatment of Acne: *Garciniamangostana* Linn

Panupon Khumsupan
and Wandee Gritsanapan[*]
Department of Pharmacognosy,
Faculty of Pharmacy, Mahidol University,
Bangkok, Thailand

Abstract

Acne vulgaris is a skin disease occurring at the cutaneous layer. It is characterized by inflammatory or non-inflammatory lesions due to the overproduction and blockage of sebum and keratinous debris in sebaceous follicles. This accumulation acts as a precursor of acne lesions called microcomedo and is highly susceptible to bacterial infection, namely *Propionibacterium acnes* and *Staphylococcus epidermidis*. Many Thai traditional herbal medicines have been recognized as effective acne treatment, including turmeric (*Curcuma longa* Linn.), Centella (*Centellaasiatica* (L.) Urb.), *Chromolaena odorata* (L.) R. M. King and H. Rob., *Houttuyniac ordata* Thunb., *Senna alata* (L.) Roxb., *Melaleuca*

---
[*]Corresponding author, E-mail: wandeegrit@yahoo.co.th.

alternifolia (Maiden and Betche) Cheel., and mangosteen (*Garcinia mangostana* Linn.). Searching for an alternative treatment has been a paramount focus in the medical field due to antibiotic resistance. Traditional medicine also has its advantage of lower side effects and abundant availability. Many traditional medicines have been under intense scrutiny for such purpose and one of the most effective herbs is mangosteen. Many researchers have reported its antimicrobial property, especially against *P. acnes* and *S. epidermidis*, and its anti-inflammatory and antioxidant properties. Due to these combinatorial properties, mangosteen and many herbal medicines with similar properties would be effective candidates to the treatment of acne. Mangosteen or *Garcinia mangostana* Linn. of the family Guttiferae is one of the most consumed fruits and distributed widely in the countries in the tropical zone. Because of its sweet and delicious taste, it is the economic fruit especially of the countries in the South East Asia. Many chemical compounds in mangosteen are responsible for its medicinal properties and the one that is present in the highest amount is α-mangostin, extracted from the rind and is especially abundant in the ripe rind. Mangosteen extract has been more popularly utilized in the cosmetic industries due to the fact that it is able to inhibit acne causing bacteria including *P. acnes* (MIC 7.81μg/mL and MBC 31.25μg/mL) and *S. epidermidis* (MIC 15.63μg/mL and MBC 31.25μg/mL). Many other xanthones, tannins and phenols, which contribute to the antioxidant and anti-inflammatory activities, can also be found in mangosteen.

Introduction

Acne vulgaris is a common skin disease affecting more than 85% of the population. It is especially prevalent in teenagers and usually resolves in the mid 20's for the majority of the patients. However, it is not limited to only teenagers since infant and adult acne could also be found, though not as common. Due to its location of occurrence, mostly on the face, neck, chest, and back, the problem of acne often deals with patient's self-esteem, social side effects, and consequently, the quality of life. Although acne does not have direct impacts on the overall health of the patient, the emotional and psychological effects, as severe as suicidal thoughts and suicide itself, could be profound [1-3].

Acne vulgaris is alesion characterized by the formation of comedones, papules, pustules, nodules, and resulting scars. The microcomedones include the open comedones or the blackheads, and the closed comedones or the white heads. Papules and pustules are inflamed comedo due to the hypercolonization of *Propionibacterium acnes*, gram-positive bacillus. Nodules, or more commonly known as cysts, are highly inflamed and deep pustules, and often accompanied by scars [2].

Acne is a disease of a pilosebaceous unit, a unit comprised of sebaceous gland, hair follicle, and the epidermis. Sebaceous glands are distributed throughout the body with the exception of the sole and palm. The number of sebaceous glands remains about the same throughout a person's life but the glands enlarge with age. The sebaceous gland's size is closely linked to genetics, and found to be regulated by androgens and steroid. Larger glands produce more sebum, greasy substance, thus consequently and possibly, more acne [1, 4].

The causes of acne are multi-factorial, including mainly genetics. Environmental factors and dietary elevate the severity of acne. It is well established that androgen plays a crucial role in acne. During puberty, local androgen mediates the production of sebum of the sebaceous gland. Other hormones also contribute to acne formation, including progesterone, glucocorticoid, estrogen, insulin, and insulin-like growth factor. Personal hygiene and some controversial dietaries such as whole milk or chocolate might inconclusively contribute to acne, but more research is needed to confirm the claim. High glycemic diet has been found to increase acne lesion but more randomized studies have to be undergone to ascertain the results [2, 4, 5].

Pathogeneses

There are four processes of acne vulgaris pathogenesis:

1. Overproduction of Sebum

The production of sebum by the sebaceous gland is primarily regulated by local androgens, mainly testosterone, which is converted to dihydrotestosterone (DHT) by isoenzyme 5-α-reductase type I. The production of these hormones and their receptors depend chiefly on the genetic makeup of an individual. During puberty, the elevated production of androgens is accompanied by the increased sebum secretion, and consequently, the blockage of the pilosebaceous follicles due to thickened epidermis [1, 2, 4].

2. Follicular Hyperkeratinization and Obstruction

Keratin is a natural structural protein found in skin. Excessive production of keratin or hyperkeratinization, influenced by genetics, intervenes with skin cell desquamation, resulting in clogging. This clogging of more dead skin cells, in addition to an increased amount of sebum, causes the blockage of follicles and the sebaceous ducts, which then leads to acne[1, 2].

3. Hypercolonization by *Propionibacterium Acnes*

P. acnes are gram-positive, anaerobic bacteria that cause acne inflammation. The anaerobic environment provided by the excess sebum in the comedones is suitable for the growth of *P. acne*. These bacteria are known to secrete lipase that can hydrolyze sebum triglycerides into comedogenic and proinflammatory free fatty acids. They also secrete proteases and hydrolases that contribute to tissue destruction. Stress proteins produced by these bacteria are further responsible for the rupture of comedones [1, 2].

4. Inflammation

P. acnes are also involved in the inflammatory response of acne by stimulating the production of cytokines like interleukins (IL-1β and IL-8) through binding to the toll-like receptors on keratinocytes. IL-1β is thought to induce in hyperkeratinization, resulting in follicular obstruction and inflammation while the other interleukins engage in a more complicated pathway involving corticotrophin releasing hormone and the production of testosterone. This, in turns, stimulates sebum production and acne. In other studies, *P. acnes* are also involved in the production of reactive oxygen species (ROS) and lysosomal enzymes through the production of neutrophil chemotactic factors, which results in disrupted follicular epithelium [1, 2].

Treatment

The current treatment of acne is to target the mentioned pathogeneses. Therefore, an array of medication is needed to:

1. Reduce sebum production either by directly or indirectly inhibiting sebaceous gland from producing sebum or inhibiting androgen's effect on the sebaceous gland (anti-androgenic agent).
2. Promote skin desquamation to reduce follicular obstruction, which will result in reduced comedo, papule, and postule counts (comedolytic agents).
3. Reduce the number of bacteria populated in the hair follicles (anti-bacterial agent).
4. Reduce inflammation and the damage to the cell (anti-inflammatory agent).

Depending on age, sex, and severity of acne, one may choose a combination of medication that target the causes of acne. Topical agents are often prescribed and have been proven to prevent and cure mild or moderate acne. The staple topical agents include retinoids, benzoyl peroxide, and an antibiotic.

Retinoids, vitamin A derivatives, promote skin desquamation and is effective in treating and preventing comedones. Consequently, this also prevents inflammation. The benefits are not without the side effects, however, as patients may experience redness and irritation. Some may experience the breakout before the clearing of the skin and the tolerance is built up after a period of application. Another side effect is photosensitivity. Patients are recommended to apply it in the evening and sun blocks should be used when sun exposure is unavoidable. Women during pregnancy are advised against retinoids since it is linked to infant malformation [1, 6].

Benzoyl peroxide is a safe and effective anticomedogenic, anti-inflammatory agent, and antimicrobial that does not produce bacterial resistance. The side effects include dryness and skin irritation but usually subside as the patient develops tolerance with frequent application. To minimize the side effect, lower concentration benzoyl peroxide may be recommended when start using [1, 6].

Topical antibiotics, such as clindamycin and erythromycin, act directly on the skin surface and within the follicles to decrease the number of *P. acnes* and thereby reduce inflammation. The disadvantage of topical antibiotic is the development of bacteria resistance and that is why antibiotics are usually used synergistically with retinoids, azelaic acid, and/or benzoyl peroxide [1].

Systemic treatment of acne is also available for moderate and severe cases. Oral antibiotics, such as tetracycline, oxytetracycline, doxycycline, and minocycline, can be prescribed. The efficacy of these antibacterial agent depends on its ability to inhibit the proliferation of *P. acnes* in the pillosebaceous follicles. Oral isotretinoin is a highly effective agent against acne due to its ability to decrease sebum production, reduce colonization by *P. acnes* and inflammation. However, its use is restricted to prescription because of its severe side effects, teratogenesis, hepatitis, and hyperlipidaemia [1].

Lasers and light therapy are another promising option to treating acne with minimal side effects, which include erythema and mild swelling. By targeting the causes of acne, *P. acnes* and sebaceous gland, lasers have become an increasingly popular and effective choice for treating lesions, inflammation, and even scarring. A range of visible and infrared lights are available for coping with different aspects of acne [7].

Anti-Acne Medicinal Plants

Nowadays, the use of medicinal plants has become more advisable and preferable due to its less hazardous nature and lower side effects. The search for new and alternative medicinal plants, especially those with antibiotic activity, for the treatment of diseases has been a central focus. New antibiotics have to be constantly developed since bacterial resistance is recurring, rendering current antibiotic less effective [8]. Many medicinal plants, ethnologically utilized or randomly screened due to its potential aptitude to reduce inflammation or restrict the proliferation of acne-inducing bacteria, are discussed with more detailed emphasis on mangosteen (*Garcinia mangostana* Linn.).

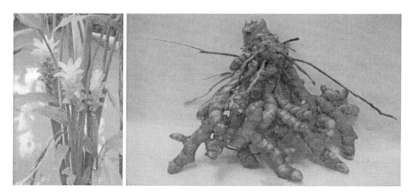

Figure 1. Turmeric (*Curcuma longa* Linn., Family Zingiberaceae) leaf, flower and rhizome.

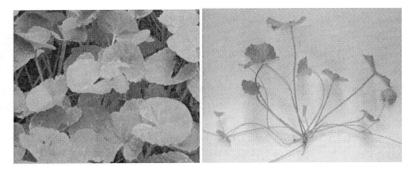

Figure 2. Centella (*Centellaasiatica* (L.) Urb.), Family Umbelliferae) leaf, and whole plant.

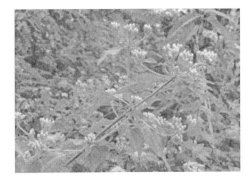

Figure 3. *Chromolaena odorata* (L.)R. M. King and H. Rob. (Asteraceae) or Siam weed leaf, stem, and flower.

Turmeric (Thai name, Kamin Chan) is the rhizome of *Curcuma longa* Linn. (Figure 1), a popular medicinal plant of Thailand and Asian countries. The rhizome contains essential oil comprising of several monoterpines and sesquiterpines such as zingiberine, ar-, α- and β-turmerone; and yellow curcuminoids pigments, which are curcumin, demethoxycurcumin and bisdemethoxycurcumin [9]. Standard of ASEAN Herbal Medicine recommend that standard turmeric powder should contain not less than 6% v/w of volatile oil and 5% w/w of total curcuminoids[10] while WHO recommended not less than 4% v/w and 3% w/w, respectively [11]. The turmeric essential oil is active for inhibiting dermatophytes, and curcuminoids are potent antioxidants and anti-inflammatory agents [12]. Staple in both the kitchen and Ayurvedic formulations, turmeric is well known for its skin benefits. With the properties ranging from anti-tumor, anti-oxidation, anti-bacteria, anti-inflammation, anti-fungi [13], and recently discovered anti-amyloid [14], it has been under an intense scrutiny by the scientific community for the last decade. Owing to the major curcuminoid, curcumin, the anti-inflammatory and anti-oxidant properties [15] are especially effective when it comes to treating acne and lesions. This is achieved by suppressing reactive oxygen species (ROS) induced by *P. acnes*. A clinical study in a hospital in Thailand in 1995 reported the effectiveness of turmeric against acne lesions. When applying turmeric powder directly on a lesion, it could reduce inflammation as well as the size, especially that of papules, pustules, and nodules [16].

Described as the "foremost" herb within the anti-aging realm, *Centellaasiatica* (Asiatic pennywort; Thai name, Bua-bok) (Figure 2) has been utilized in the cosmeceutical Ayuravedic medicine for centuries. The main use in the acne treatment is focused on treating scars and wounds from acne because of its potent anti-oxidant and collagen synthetic properties [13]. The major phytochemical constituents responsible for its activities are pentacyclic triterpenes called centelloids. Predominantly, four active triterpene derivatives, cassoside, madecassic acid, asiaticoside, and asiatic acid, possess pharmaceutical properties [17]. Madecassocide has been known for its wound-healing effects while asiaticoside induces type I collagen synthesis and gene expression of human fibroblast [18]. Besides coping with the senescence process, this "potential cure-all" is also recommended for an array of skin and other diseases, including leprosy, lupus, varicose, ulcers, eczema, psoriasis, diarrhea, fever, amenorrhea, in addition to relieving anxiety and improving cognition [19].

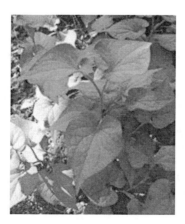

Figure 4. *Houttuyniac ordata* Thunb. (Family Saururaceae) leaf.

Chromolaena odorata or Siam weed (Thai name, Sap suea) (Figure 3) is a perennial scandent or semi-woody shrub native to Central and South America and spreads throughout the tropical and subtropical areas of the world [20]. Formally known as *Eupatorium odoratum* Linn., this medicinal herb has been extensively used as a blood coagulating and wound-healing agent. The chemical constituents were reported to be volatile oil, phenolic compounds, tannins, saponins, terpenoids, alkaloids, and flavonoids which were the main component [21-24]. Several flavonoids such as kaempferol-4'-methylether, naringenin-4'-methylether (isosakuranetin) and 4',5,6,7- tetramethoxy-flavone were isolated from *C. odorata* extracts [25, 26]. The extract has been demonstrated clinically and histologically to stimulate the formation of granulation tissue and wound re-epithelialization [27]. It also inhibited the contraction of collagen lattices by normal human dermal fibroblasts *in vitro* [28]. The treatment of acne using *C. odorata* is mostly clinically unexplored although there have been reports of its anti-bacterial and antioxidant activities. The extract of the leaves was able to inhibit the growth of bacteria – *Pseudomonas aeroginosa, Escherichia coli, Staphylococcus aureus,* and *Neisseria gonorrhea*. The MIC and MBC against *P. acnes* were 0.625 and 1.25 mg/ml, respectively [29]. The concentration range of 50- 800 µg/ml showed significant protection against hydrogen peroxide and superoxide radicals on cultured fibroblasts and keratinocytes [28].

Houttuyniac ordata (Thai name, PhluKhao) (Figure 4) is a perennial herb in which the whole plant has distinctively fishy taste. It is traditionally used for a diuretic and disinfectant for urinary tract. The whole plant contains volatile oil comprising aldehydes, N-methyl nomylketone, and flavonoids, such as quercitrin and rutin [30, 31]. Like *Chromolaena odorata, Houttuyniac ordata*'s potential against acne is yet to be pioneered. Its potential against acne lies within two essential activities: anti-acne-inducing bacterial, *P. acnes*, and anti-inflammatory activities. The anti-inflammatory mechanism is accomplished through the binding to cyclooxygenase (COX) enzymes to prevent the production of prostaglandins [32]. Volatile oils were believed to be responsible for this activity. Its potency against bacteria associating with skin diseases is also comparable to that of *Garcinia mangostana*, a well-known and preferable choice of herbal medicine against acne. The MIC and MBC were 0.039 mg/ml and 2.5 mg/ml against *P. acnes*, respectively, while the MIC against *S. epidermidis* was 1.25 mg/ml [29].

Senna alata (Candelabra bush or Ringworm bush) (Figure 5) is known in Thai as Chumhetthet.

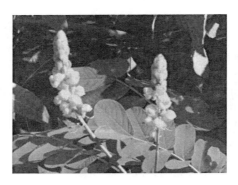

Figure 5. *Senna alata* (L.) Roxb. (Family Leguminosae-Caesalpinioideae) leaf and flower.

It is a native plant of South America and can be found widely in tropical region. *S. alata*is a medicinal plant of which the leaves have long been used as antifungal drugs. It is one of the plants recommended to be used in primary health care in Thailand. It is also known for its laxative property due to the abundance of anthraquinones such as rhein and aloe-emodin, both in aglycone and glycoside forms. According to the Standard of ASEAN Herbal Medicine, *S. alata* leaves should contain not less than 0.5% dry weight of total hydroxyanthracene derivatives calculated as rhein-8-glucoside [10]. Total anthraquinones content in the leaves of *Senna alata* is more extensively used to treat skin conditions. Crushed leaves and decoction have been ethnologically used to treat an array of skin diseases, including dermatitis, skin rash, eczema, and athlete's foot. Other biological activities, such as antibacterial, antiviral, and anti-inflammatory activities, are due to the presence of steroids and flavonoids, like stigmasterol and kaempferol [33]. The extract was also moderately active against both *S. epidermidis* and *P. acnes*, with the MIC and MBC of *P. acnes* being 0.625 mg/ml and 2.5 mg/ml, respectively [29].

Melaleuca Alternifolia (Maiden and Betche) Cheel. (Tea Tree) (Family Myrtaceae)

Melaleuca alternifolia (Maiden and Betche) Cheel. (Family Myrtaceae) or tea tree is an Australian native plant used largely for its antimicrobial properties. The plant is an evergreen shrub of 5 to 8 m in height with narrow, 4 cm, needle-like leaves and releases a distinctive aroma when crushed. The indigenous people of Australia have used tea tree oil from crushed leaves as a traditional remedy for coughs and colds, as well as wounds and skin conditions. The essential oil extracted by steam distillation of the leaves and terminal branches of this plant has been used for almost 100 years in Australia but is now available worldwide including in Thailand. The yield of oil is typically 1 to 2% wet weight. Tea tree oil was first used in surgery and dentistry in the mid-1920s. Its healing properties were also used during World War II for skin injuries. Tea tree oil is composed of terpene hydrocarbons, mainly monoterpenes, sesquiterpenes, and their associated alcohols [34]. Renowned for its potency against acne, tea tree oil has been included in several commercial products. Its 5% essential oil has been clinically compared to benzoyl peroxide and proven to be more effective in terms of reduction of total acne lesions and acne severity index [35, 36]. Monoterpenes and sesquiterpenes hydrocarbons and their alcohols (alpha-terpineol, terpinen-4-ol, alpha-pinene, among many others) are responsible for its anti-inflammatory (through the reduction of histamine) and antimicrobial activities and are used against yeasts, fungi, and bacteria [37]. The MIC against *P. acnes* and *S. epidermidis* were 0.31- 0.63 and 0.63-1.23% v/v, respectively [38].

Mangosteen (*Garcinia mangostana* Linn.) (Family Guttiferae) (Thai name, Mangkhut) (Figure 6) is one of the most useful plants with many medicinal properties and has been under intense scrutiny for the past years. The origin of mangosteen is unclear but believed to be first domesticated in Thailand or Burma [39]. Mangosteen is widely grown in the tropical regions, especially South East Asia, and known by many names including palo de cruz in Spanish, and mangostanier in French [40]. Titled "the queen of fruits," mangosteen aril has juicy, sweet taste and mild pleasant aroma [41]. Although the aril has been used as nutraceutical supplement for its antioxidant activity, the exocarp or the rind is usually the byproduct from the edible aril part.

Mangosteen rind has traditionally been used to treat abdominal pain, diarrhea, dysentery, skin infection, suppuration, and chronic ulcer [42]. Scientific evidences have demonstrated that, moreover, mangosteen rind possesses many biological activities such as antioxidant, anti-inflammatory, antibacterial, and potentially antiviral activities. These biological activities owe to many polyphenolic compounds, such as tannins, flavonoids, and xanthones. One of the major xanthones being heavily studied now is α-mangostin (IUPAC name: 3,6,8-Trihydroxy-2-methoxy-1,7-bis(3-methylbut-2-enyl)xanthen-9-one) [43-45]. Studies have confirmed the inhibitory effects of α-mangostin to *P. acnes* and *S. epidermis*, which are bacteria that trigger inflammation and cause acne. Consequently, mangosteen rind extract and α-mangostin have been exploited more recently in the cosmetic industry [29].

Mangosteen rind also comprises of many other chemical constituents including the less abundant β- and γ- mangostin, and garcinones. This review focuses on the utilization and the chemical components, as well as the biological properties of the mangosteen rind.

Distribution of mangosteen

Mangosteen has spread throughout many tropical countries, namely Sri Lanka, India, Countries in Central and South America, Australia, and some states in the USA. A large scale production of mangosteen locates in countries in the Southeast Asia such as Vietnam, Burma, Cambodia, Malaysia, Indonesia, the Philippines, and especially Thailand, where more than 11,000 ha (in 2000) were dedicated to cultivation [39, 46].

Although the origin is unclear, *G. mangostana* is believed to originate from the Sunda Islands and the Moluccas. It was introduced in India in 1881, but only survived in limited areas. The introduction reached Central America in the early 1900's, but only a few trees survived in the Panama Canal zone, Puerto Rico, Jamaica, Dominica, and Cuba [39, 46].

The introduction to the United States occurred in the early 1900's when the US Department of Agriculture obtained the seeds from Java. The early trial happened in Hawaii but failed due to soil and climate. Other potential states included California and Florida. *G. mangostana* could not tolerate the climate in the former, but was somewhat successful in the latter despite the cold winter [46].

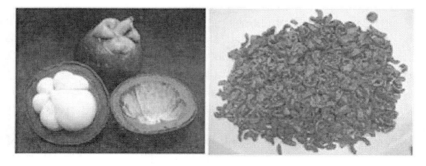

Figure 6. Mangosteen (*Garcinia mangostana* Linn.) (Family Guttiferae) fruit and dried rind.

Extract Preparation

Extraction of the medicinal plant raw material is an essential step to obtain the bioactive components qualitatively and quantitatively. The ideal method of extraction should be inexpensive, rapid, consistent, and easy to perform repeatedly. Therefore, the most appropriate method of extraction should be identified before the analysis of chemical constituents.

Depending on the bioactive compounds, ranging from the more hydrophobic terpenoids and essential oils to the less hydrophobic flavonoids and phenols, the extraction method from different plants can vary. For instance, if that compound is tolerant to heat, Soxhlet extraction could potentially be ideal. Percolation or maceration would be more appropriate for more easily degraded compounds, keeping in mind that these methods require more solvents and time [47]. With regards to obtaining crude extracts from *G. mangostana* rind, Soxhlet extraction with 95% ethanol gave the highest yield (26.60 %w/w of dried powder, 13.51 %w/w of α-mangostin, 24.83 gallic acid equivalent (GAE)/100 g extract of total phenolic compounds, 41.94 g tannic acid equivalent (TAE)/100 g extract of total tannins, and 11.93 g quercetin equivalent (QE)/100 g extract of total flavonoids. However, further investigation using 70% and 50% ethanol in addition to 95% ethanol found that 70% and 50% ethanol gave higher yields of crude extracts, total phenolics, and total tannins, but lower yields of α-mangostin and total flavonoids. Due to the more polar nature of 50% and 70% ethanol, they could easily dissolve more polar compounds like phenolics and tannins, but less of α-mangostin and total flavonoids. Soxhlet extraction with 95% ethanol yielded higher amount of α-mangostin (13.5% w/w) and total flavonoids (11.93 g QE/100 g extract). This result strongly correlated to the antioxidant and antibacterial activities. Since tannins and phenolic compounds promoted better radical scavenging activity, Soxhlet extraction with 70% and 50% ethanol were more effective for the preparation against free radicals (EC_{50}: 13.39 and 12.84 µg/ml, respectively). On the other hand, Soxhlet extraction with 95% ethanol possessed better bacteriostatic activity due to the abundance of α-mangostin (MIC of against *P. acnes* of 7.81 µg/ml for 95% ethanol and 15.63 µg/ml for both 50% and 70% ethanol extracts) [46, 48].

Another method that was looked into was ultrasonic extraction because it was more time-efficient. However, this method gave lower yield than Soxhlet extraction, possibly because of oxidation and degradation of bioactive compounds during the process of sonication. Therefore, Soxhlet extraction was the most appropriate method for extracting mangosteen rind. However, depending on the purpose of the extraction, one could choose 50%, 70%, or 95% ethanol in the extraction process [46].

To extract and purify α-mangostin, Soxhlet extraction with dichloromethane was preferred because of the more nonpolar nature of dichloromethane that was more specifically suitable to extract α-mangostin. After obtaining the crude extract, the isolation could be done by silica gel column chromatography, eluting with hexane, hexane/dichloromethane, dichloromethane/ethyl acetate with increasing polarity. The reported yield was 32.76 mg α-mangostin from 100 g of fruit rind extract. Purified α-mangostin compound should be amorphous yellow powder with the melting point of $180°$ – $182°C$. The Rf value should be equal to that of the α-mangostin reference standard, which is 0.40 [46, 49].

Stability of *G. Mangostana* Extract

The stability test was done by keeping *G. mangostana* crude 95% ethanol extract in amber glass vial and aluminum foil bag in 3 different temperatures (4-8 $°C$, 25-28$°C$, and 45$°C$) for 4 months. The physical changes were observed every month and it was found that crude extracts kept in 4-8$°C$ remained physically unchanged. The appearance of the crude extracts in the other 2 conditions changed into brown semi-solid, instead of yellow-brown fine powder [50]. The amount of α-mangostin from each condition was also evaluated every month for 4 months by validated HPLC. Assuming that at day 0, the α-mangostin content was at 100%, the α-mangostin content remained relatively unchanged (ranged from 90.20 to 101.23%) for all conditions after 4 months. It could be concluded that storage temperature up to 4 months had no effect on the α-mangostin content in the extract [50].

Biological stability was evaluated by testing the crude extract of each storage condition against bacteria *P. acne* and *S. epidermidis*, and performing DPPH radical assay. To test for the antibacterial activity, broth microdilution was performed, and found that at day 0, the MIC and MBC for *P. acnes* were 7.81 µg/ml, and 15.63 µg/ml, respectively. For *S. epidermidis*, the MIC value was 15.63 µg/ml and MBC value was 31.25 µg/ml. After 1,2,3, and 4 months, the antibacterial activity in the amber glass vial and aluminum foil in 4, 25, and 25$°C$ were relatively unchanged [50].

For the antiradical activity, the DPPH scavenging assay was performed. Similar to the result of the antibacterial activity, the antiradical activity remained relatively unchanged. The initial $1/EC_{50}$ value was 0.0790 w/w. The change of antiradical activity of the extracts in the foil bag and the amber glass vial after 4 months in 3 different temperatures were in the range of 96.98 to 103.40% of the initial activity. These results proved that storage temperature (up to 4 months) and the type of container had very little impact on the antiradical and antibacterial activities of *G. mangostana* rind extract [50].

Standardization of *Garcinia Mangostana* Extract

The amount of total phenolic compounds in crude extract and dry powder from different provinces in Thailand were compared. The average content of phenolic compounds in the extract was 22.33 +/- 3.25 g and 6.13 +/- 1.69 g in dry powder (GAE/100 g). The average content of total phenolic compounds in the samples from different locations was not significantly different (p > 0.05) [49].

Similar to phenolic compound contents, the average total tannins, analyzed by protein precipitation method, from different locations was not significantly different (p > 0.05). The average content of total tannins was 36.38 +/- 8.46 g in crude extract and 10.11 +/- 3.83 g in dry powder (TAE/100 g) [48].

By aluminum chloride colorimetry, the average content of total flavonoids was 4.13 +/- 1.10 g in crude extract and 0.80 +/- 0.16 g in dry powder (QE/100g). The average content of total flavonoids in samples collected from different locations was not significantly different (p> 0.05) [46].

Method Validation of the Quantitative Analysis of Active Compound alpha-Mangostin

Method validation is the process that confirms the suitability of the procedures and also an indication of the reliability and consistency of the analysis method. Method validation of α-mangostin has been done in TLCdensitometer and HPLC. Both procedures have their advantages and can act as a basis or guidance for further standardization of α-mangostin obtained from mangosteen rind extracts. The comparison between both methods is shown below [51, 52].

Table 1. Comparison of HPLC and TLC-densitometry validation methods

Quantitative parameters	HPLC	TLC-densitometry
Linear range	10-200 µg/ml (100-2000 ng)	100–500 ng/spot
Regression equation	y = 33674x - 7244.7	y = 31.469x + 2359.4
Correlation coefficient (r^2)	0.9999	0.999
LOQ	0.17 µg/ml (1.7 ng)	100 ng
LOD	0.06 µg/ml (0.6 ng)	40 ng
Inter-day and intraday precision (expressed as % RSD)	Less than 2%	Less than 2%
Accuracy (% recovery)	105.10, 95.00, and 99.93% with standard deviation being 1.21, 1.81, and 1.51%, respectively	102.37, 97.72, and 98.37% with standard deviation being 3.46, 4.82, and 3.09%, respectively

Being a more modern and complex method, HPLC produced a more desirable data, having better LOQ, LOD, accuracy, and precision. However, operation of HPLC is discouraging due to a more complex and expensive system. Although being less reproducible, TLC-densitometry could be desirable in cases where time was a restraint, since it could screen many samples simultaneously [51, 52].

Biological Activities

Antimicrobial Activity

Many research studies have undergone to investigate the effectiveness of mangosteen extracts against microorganisms, especially acne causing bacteria *P. acnes* and *S. epidermidis*. The MIC values of extract against *P. acnes* and *S. epidermidis* were found to be 13.02 and 23.44 µg/mL, respectively while the average MBC values were 15.63 and 83.33 µg/mL, respectively. However, isolated α-mangostin proved to be more effective against *P. acnes* and *S. epidermidis* with the MIC and MBC value of 1.95 µg/ml for *P. acnes* and 3.91 µg/ml for *S. epidermidis* [53]. From this finding, we could infer that α-mangostin, a xanthone, was an active antibacterial component and could be used as a marker for *G. mangostana* extracts and products. Consistently, Chomnawang et al. (2005) showed that *G. mangostana* extract, the most effective antibacterial extract out of the 13 medicinal plants tested, produced strong inhibition zones against *P. acnes* and *S. epidermidis* [29].

Suksamrarn et al. (2003) found that α-mangostin, β-mangostin, and garcinone B extracted from the seeds, arils, and fruit hulls of *G. mangostana* had a strong inhibitory effect against *Mycobacterium tuberculosis*. These prenylated xanthones had the MIC of 6.25 µg/ml (54). Additionally, *G. mangostana* pericarb extract had an inhibitory effect and could stimulate phagocytic cells to kill intracellular bacteria like *Salmonella enteritidis* [55].

The inhibitory effect of *G. mangostana* extracts was also tested on vancomycin resistant *Enterococci* and methicillin-resistant *Staphylococcus aureus*. It was found that the active component responsible for the effect was α-mangostin, and had the MIC of 1.57 to 12.5 µg/ml, which was greater than that of vancomycin (3.13 to 6.25 µg/ml). α-Mangostin was also found to have partial synergism with antibiotics such as ampicillin and minocyclin, boosting their antibacterial activity [56, 57]. Voravuthikunchai [2005] confirmed that *G. mangostana* aqueous and ethanolic extracts were one of the most effective inhibitory agent against hospital isolated, methicillin-resistant *S. aureus*, with the MIC of 0.05-0.4 mg/ml [58].

Antioxidant Activity

Radicals are byproducts from our cells from producing energy. Although it is damaging to cells, our body has a way to regulate and rid of radicals by producing enzymes such as superoxide dismutase. However, as we grow older, our body is not as capable to produce enough antiradical enzymes to cope with this problem. Taking supplement is often one of the ways to help our body maintain its normal function.

It is well accepted that natural compounds like phenolic compounds including flavonoids, phenolic acids, and tannins in medicinal plants are effective against free radicals. Their redox ability acting as reducing agents, hydrogen donators, singlet oxygen quenchers, and their metal chelating ability make them superb antioxidant candidates. Pothitirat et al. (2010) [48] claimed that there was a correlation between antiradical activity and the content of total flavonoids and α-mangostin content. By DPPH scavenging and NBT reduction assays, they concluded that phenolic compounds and tannin in *G. mangostana* rind were responsible for free radical scavenging property and were able to reduce reactive oxygen species production [48, 53, 59]. Chin (2008) isolated and identified 16 compounds from *G. mangostana* dichloromethane rind extract using bioactivity guided fractionation. Utilizing quinine reductase-induction assay and hydroxyl radical antioxidant assay, they found that γ-mangostin exhibited a high hydroxyl radical-scavenging activity with the IC_{50} of 0.20 µg/ml [60].

Through its antioxidant activity, α-mangostin may lead to the prevention of atheroscorosis and myocardial infarction. Because of the antioxidant activity, α-mangostin prevented lipid peroxidation induced in rats by isoproterenol. After oral administration of α-mangostin (200 mg/kg body weight) for 6 days prior the administration of isoproterenol and 2 days along with isoproterenol, rats in the experimental groups were found to be more peroxidation-resistant compared to the controlled group [61].

Anti-Inflammatory Activity

Inflammation is an innate immune response of an organism to the pathogen and often results in swelling, heat, pain, redness, and consequently, loss of function. Many biological mediators, such as nitric oxide, cyclooxygenase (COX), histamine, and interleukin-1 alpha (IL-1α), are involved in the process. Inhibition of these mediators or the rate-determining enzymes is the crucial key to reduce inflammation. Many studies have shown that constituents in mangosteen rind exhibit potent anti-inflammatory property through various mechanisms.

Through ELISA, the crude ethanolic extract of *G. mangostana* was found to be effective in the treatment of inflammation stimulated by heat-killed *P. acnes*. *G. mangostana* extract (50 µg/ml) was able to significantly reduce the production of TNF-α, a pro-inflammatory cytokines, at 94.59%. The dose-dependent inhibitory effect was the highest among medicinal herbs tested (*G. mangostana, E. odoratum, H. cordata, and S. siame*) [59].

Gamma-mangostin, one of the xanthones in the fruit rind of *G. mangostana*, was found to be an active anti-inflammatory due to its antagonistic effect to serotonin 2 (5-HT$_2$) receptor. The mechanism responsible for this effect was investigated using NG 108-15 cells treated with γ-mangostin or a 5-HT$_2$ receptor antagonist. Semi-quantitative RT-PCR was used to monitor the level of mRNA receptors. They revealed that γ-mangostin enhanced the expression of 5-HT$_{2A/2C}$, muscarinnic, histamine, and brady kinin receptor mRNA, inferring that this xanthone has antagonistic effects [62].

Alpha-mangostin and γ-mangostin were able to exert its anti-inflammatory activity by other means as well. In the study by Bumrungpert et al., (2009) they came to the conclusion that both xanthones were able to suppress the inflammation induced by lipopolysaccharide (LPS) in human adipocytes. Xanthones, especially γ-mangostin, lowered the expression of inflammatory genes, including tumor necrosis factor-α, interleukin (IL)-1β, IL-6, IL-8, monocyte chemoattractant protein-1, and Toll-like receptor-2 [63].

To elucidate the mechanism of inflammatory inhibition by α-mangostin and γ-mangostin, Chen et al. utilized Raw 264.7 cells. They proposed that xanthones, specifically α-mangostin and γ-mangostin, exerted the anti-inflammatory effect by inhibiting the expression of inducible nitric oxide synthase (iNOS) and COX-2. Through this *in vivo* study, they proved that both xanthones could reduce NO production in a dose-dependent manner with the IC$_{50}$ being 12.4 and 10.1 μM for α-mangostin and γ-mangostin, respectively. In addition, they could also significantly reduce PGE$_2$ production with γ-mangostin being more efficient. The reduction of NO was accomplished by inhibiting the expression of iNOS, but not the iNOS activity. Unlike iNOS, COX-2 expression was not inhibited but the activity of COX-2 was [64].

Another set of experiment to show the anti-inflammatory activity of xanthones was to induce edema by carrageenan in mice hand paw. Alpha-mangostin was more efficient than sulindac, the positive control, at inhibiting paw adema at 3 h and 5 h, which referred to the initial phase involved in the release of histamine and serotonin and the second phase involved in the release of prostaglandin-like substances. However, γ-mangostin did not significantly inhibit the edema [64].

Anti-Tumor Activity

Garcinia mangostana also possesses the anti-tumoral effect. The study was done on rats that were injected with 1,2-dimethylhydrazine (DMH) (40 mg/kg body weight, once a week for 2 weeks) to induce colon carcinogenesis. The rats in the experimental groups were fed with 0.02% and 0.5% crude α-mangostin starting 1 week prior to the injection of DMH for 5 weeks. After the experiment was terminated, they found that rats that were fed with α-mangostin developed less or no aberrant crypt foci in a dose dependent manner compared to the controlled groups [65]. The mechanism of colorectal cancer inhibition was found to be caspase-independent and involved the release of endonuclease-G and the expression of microRNA-143, causing apoptosis and cytotoxicity against colon cancer DLD-1 cells [66]. This suggested that α-mangostin was a potent chemotherapeutic agent in this short-term colon carcinogenesis bioassay system and could potentially be developed into tumor suppressing medicine.

Another research study was done to investigate the apoptotic effect of *G. mangostana* pericarp methanolic extract on breast cancer cell line (SKBR3). They discovered that the *G. mangostana* extract showed an antiproliferative effect (ED_{50} of 9.25 +/- 0.64 µg/ml) determined by the morphological changes and oligonucleosomal DNA fragments in a dose dependent and exposure time dependent manner [67]. The antiproliferative mechanism of *G. mangostana* extract against breast cancer cell line was explained by Balunas (2008) using a noncellular, enzyme-based microsomal aromatase inhibition assay. Aromatase was the key enzyme that promoted the production of estrogens and consequently induced certain breast cancers. Xanthones in the extract – garcinone D, garcinone E, α-mangostin, and γ-mangostin (the most potent) – were active aromatase inhibitory compounds [68].

Alpha-mangostin could also induce apoptosis in HL60 cells through the mitochondrial pathway. They found that 6 xanthones from the *G. mangostana* rind extract displayed growth inhibitory effects, especially α-mangostin that showed the complete inhibition at 10 µM [69]. The treatment of α-mangostin on the HL60 cell did not interfere with the bcl-2 family proteins and activation of MAP kinases. However, the potency decreased when replacing the hydroxyl group by the methoxy group. This finding concluded that α-mangostin was a plausible chemotherapeutic candidate [70].

Using the MTT method, Ho et al. (2002) showed that garcinone E, one of the xanthones derived from *G. mangostana* rind, possessed the cytotoxic effects on 14 different human cancer cell lines including 6 hepatoma cell lines and other gastric and lung cancer cell lines. While chemotherapy had been mostly ineffective, garcinone E could potentially be beneficial in the treatment of many types of cancer [71].

The recent study utilized more than just pericarps of *G. mangostana* but also the stems and roots, which led to the discovery of new xanthone (2,8-dihydroxy-6-methoxy-5-(3-methylbut-2-enyl)-xanthone) that were potentially chemotherapeutic. The research led by Ee et al. (2008) took advantage of the hexane extracts of the stems and roots of *G. mangostana* anti-cancer activity and tested it against the CEM-SS cell line. They found that α-mangostin, mangostanol, and garcinone D had significant activities with IC$_{50}$ of 5.5, 9.6, and 3.2 µg/ml, respectively [72].

Conclusion

Accounting for more than 30% of the dermatologist visits, acne vulgaris is a skin disease that has been receiving enormous attention. Although it is not directly life-threatening, its chronicity from adolescence to adulthood is detrimental to self-esteem; and therefore, deteriorates the patient's health and emotion. Because of this, the discovery of more anti-acne medication is of the essence. Ideally, the medication should treat the four pathogeneses of acne and further prevent recurrence. A multitude of medication is usually employed because a single medication is incapable to cope with all four pathogeneses. The medication that encounters the most problem is antibacterial drugs due to antibiotic resistance. Clindamycin and erythromycin, the current antibiotic prescribed nowadays, are being rendered less effective, especially when the patient needs to take them for other more severe infection.

Medicinal herbs offer safer and exceptionally effective alternatives to synthetic drugs. Many ethnologically used herbs, such as *Curcuma longa*, *Centellaasiatica*, *Chromaolaena odorata*, *Houttuynia cordata*, *Senna alata*, *Melaleuca alternifolia*, and *Garcinia mangostana*, have been utilized in skin treatment and could potentially provide the insight to the leading compound in the management of acne. Some of these herbs, like *G. mangostana*, *M. alternifolia*, and *H. cordata*, are not only antibacterial, they are also antioxidative and anti-inflammatory. Due to its exemplarily potent antiacne property, phytochemical constituents in *G. mangostana* have been employed in cosmeceutical industry.

Since the past few decades, the center of attention has slowly shifted to the usage of medicinal herbs because of the realization of the vast benefits and minimal risks of herbs over synthetic medicines. Due to a wide array of plant species, screening for pharmaceutical activities require time, funding, and resources. We think that medicinal herbs deserve more attention since they endow us with great potential to preventing and treating acne, as well as many other diseases.

Acknowledgments

We would like to thank Mr. IthipolIthiamnuaypan, Department of Pharmacognosy, Faculty of Pharmacy, Mahidol University, for the pictures. We would also like to thank Dr. WeerayutPothitirat, Faculty of Pharmacy, Siam University, for his guidance and information.

References

[1] Shaw L, Kennedy C. The treatment of acne. *Pediatrics and Child Health*. 2007; 17(10):385-9.
[2] Nguyen R, Su J. Treatment of acne vulgaris. *Pediatrics and Child Health*. 2010; 21(3):119-25.
[3] Hedden SL, Davidson S, Smith CB. Cause and effect: The relationship between acne and self-esteem in adolescent years. *The Journal for Nurse Practitioners*. 2008;4(8):595-600.
[4] Arora MK, Yadav A, Saini V. Role of hormones in acne vulgaris. *Clin. Biochem*. 2011 Sep;44(13):1035-40.
[5] Bowe WP, Joshi SS, Shalita AR. Diet and acne. *J. Am. Acad. Dermatol*. 2010 Jul;63(1):124-41.
[6] Thiboutot D, Gollnick H, Bettoli V, Dreno B, Kang S, Leyden JJ, et al. New insights into the management of acne: an update from the Global Alliance to Improve Outcomes in Acne group. *J. Am. Acad. Dermatol*. 2009 May;60(5 Suppl):S1-50.
[7] Bhardwaj SS, Rohrer TE, Arndt K. Lasers and light therapy for acne vulgaris. *Semin. Cutan. Med. Surg*. 2005 Jun;24(2):107-12.
[8] Swanson JK. Antibiotic resistance of Propionibacterium acnes in acne vulgaris. *Dermatol. Nurs*. 2003 Aug;15(4):359-62.
[9] Pothitirat W, Gritsanapan W. Variation of bioactive components in Curcuma longa in Thailand. *Current Science*. 2006;91(10):1397-400.
[10] ASEAN Countries. Standard of ASEAN herbal medicine. Jakarta: AksaraBuana Printing; 1993. p. 14.
[11] WHO Organization. WHO monographs on selected medicinal plants. Geneva1999. p. 1.
[12] Gritsanapan W, Pothitirat W. Traditional herbs for healthcare - A case history with turmeric. In: Houghton PJ, Mukherjee PK, editors.

Evaluation of Herbal Medicinal Products. London: the Pharmaceutical Press, London; 2009. p. 18.
[13] Kanlayavattanakul M, Lourith N. Therapeutic agents and herbs in topical application for acne treatment. *Int. J. Cosmet. Sci.* 2011 Aug;33(4):289-97.
[14] Yang F, Lim GP, Begum AN, Ubeda OJ, Simmons MR, Ambegaokar SS, et al. Curcumin inhibits formation of amyloid beta oligomers and fibrils, binds plaques, and reduces amyloid in vivo. *J. Biol. Chem.* 2005 Feb 18;280(7):5892-901.
[15] Sharma RA, Gescher AJ, Steward WP. Curcumin: the story so far. *Eur. J. Cancer.* 2005 Sep;41(13):1955-68.
[16] Research team of Somdet-prayuparach-tatpanom hospital. A Study on anti-acne effectiveness of Turmeric. Nakornpanom 1995.
[17] Brinkhaus B, Lindner M, Schuppan D, Hahn EG. Chemical, pharmacological and clinical profile of the East Asian medical plant Centella asiatica. *Phytomedicine.* 2000 Oct;7(5):427-48.
[18] Bonte F, Dumas M, Chaudagne C, Meybeck A. Influence of asiatic acid, madecassic acid, and asiaticoside on human collagen I synthesis. *Planta Med.* 1994 Apr;60(2): 133-5.
[19] Datta HS, Paramesh R. Trends in aging and skin care: Ayurvedic concepts. *J. Ayurveda Integr. Med.* 2010 Apr;1(2):110-3.
[20] Muniappan R, Marutani M. Distribution and control of Chromolaena odorata (Asteraceae). *Micronesica Suppl.* 1991;3:103-7.
[21] Thongpraditchot S, Suvitayavat W, Temsiriririrkkul R. Effect of *Eupatorium odoratum* Linn. on vascular tone and primary irritation test. *Mahidol. J. Pharm. Sci.* 1994;21:44-9.
[22] Pisutthanan N, Liawruangrath S, Bremner JB, Liawruangrath B. Chemical constituents and biological activities of *Chromolaena odorata*. *J. Sci. Fac. Chiang Mai Univ.* 2005;32:139-48.
[23] Umukoro S, Ashorobi RB. Evaluation of the anti-inflammatory and membrane-stabilizing effects of *Eupatorium odoratum*. *Int. J. Pharm.* 2006;2:509-12.
[24] Pandith H, Thongpraditchote S, Wongkrajang Y, Gritsanapan W. *In vivo* and *in vitro* hemostatic activity of *Chromolaena odorata* leaf extract. *Pharmaceutical Biology.* 2012:In press.
[25] Naengchomnong W. Chemical constituents of *Jatrophacurcas* (Euphorbiaceae) and *Eupatorium odoratum* (Compositae). Bangkok: Mahidol University; 1989.

[26] Triratana T, Suwannuraks R, Naengchomnong W. Effect of Eupatorium odoratum on blood coagulation. *J. Med. Assoc. Thai.* 1991 May;74(5):283-7.
[27] Phan TT, Wang L, See P, Grayer RJ, Chan SY, Lee ST. Phenolic compounds of Chromolaena odorata protect cultured skin cells from oxidative damage: implication for cutaneous wound healing. *Biol. Pharm. Bull.* 2001 Dec;24(12):1373-9.
[28] Phan TT, Hughes MA, Cherry GW. Effects of an aqueous extract from the leaves of Chromolaena odorata (Eupolin) on the proliferation of human keratinocytes and on their migration in an in vitro model of reepithelialization. *Wound Repair Regen.* 2001 Jul-Aug;9(4):305-13.
[29] Chomnawang MT, Surassmo S, Nukoolkarn VS, Gritsanapan W. Antimicrobial effects of Thai medicinal plants against acne-inducing bacteria. *J. Ethnopharmacol.* 2005 Oct 3;101(1-3):330-3.
[30] Xu CJ, Liang YZ, Chau FT. Identification of essential components of Houttuynia cordata by gas chromatography/mass spectrometry and the integrated chemometric approach. *Talanta.* 2005 Nov 15;68(1):108-15.
[31] Lu HM, Liang YZ, Chen S. Identification and quality assessment of Houttuynia cordata injection using GC-MS fingerprint: a standardization approach. *J. Ethnopharmacol.* 2006 May 24;105(3):436-40.
[32] Li W, Zhou P, Zhang Y, He L. Houttuynia cordata, a novel and selective COX-2 inhibitor with anti-inflammatory activity. *J. Ethnopharmacol.* 2011 Jan 27;133(2):922-7.
[33] Hennebelle T, Weniger B, Joseph H, Sahpaz S, Bailleul F. Senna alata. *Fitoterapia.* 2009 Oct;80(7):385-93.
[34] Carson CF, Hammer KA, Riley TV. Melaleuca alternifolia (Tea Tree) oil: a review of antimicrobial and other medicinal properties. *Clin. Microbiol. Rev.* 2006 Jan;19(1): 50-62.
[35] Reuter J, Merfort I, Schempp CM. Botanicals in dermatology: an evidence-based review. *Am. J. Clin. Dermatol.* 2010;11(4):247-67.
[36] Bassett IB, Pannowitz DL, Barnetson RS. A comparative study of tea-tree oil versus benzoylperoxide in the treatment of acne. *Med. J. Aust.* 1990 Oct 15;153(8):455-8.
[37] Koh KJ, Pearce AL, Marshman G, Finlay-Jones JJ, Hart PH. Tea tree oil reduces histamine-induced skin inflammation. *Br. J. Dermatol.* 2002 Dec;147(6):1212-7.
[38] Raman A, Weir U, Bloomfield SF. Antimicrobial effects of tea-tree oil and its major components on Staphylococcus aureus, Staph. epidermidis

and Propionibacterium acnes. *Lett. Appl. Microbiol.* 1995 Oct;21(4):242-5.
[39] Lamoureux CH. Fruits. Bogor, Indonesia: International Board for Plant Genetic Resources; 1980.
[40] Mohamad BO, Rahman AM. Mangosteen: Garcinia mangostana L. Southampton, England: International Centre for Underutilised Crops; 2006.
[41] Martin FW. Durian and mangosteen. Nagy S, Shaw D, editors. CT: The AVI Publishing Company; 1980.
[42] Farnworth RN, Bunyapraphatsara N. *Garcinia mangostana* Linn. in Thai medicinal plants. Bangkok, Thailand: Prachachon Co., Ltd.; 1992.
[43] Jung HA, Su BN, Keller WJ, Mehta RG, Kinghorn AD. Antioxidant xanthones from the pericarp of Garcinia mangostana (Mangosteen). *J. Agric. Food Chem.* 2006 Mar 22;54(6):2077-82.
[44] Vieira LM, Kijjoa A. Naturally-occurring xanthones: recent developments. *Curr. Med. Chem.* 2005;12(21):2413-46.
[45] Peres V, Nagem TJ, de Oliveira FF. Tetraoxygenated naturally occurring xanthones. *Phytochemistry.* 2000 Dec;55(7):683-710.
[46] Pothitirat W. Standardization and development of anti-acne preparation of *Garcinia mangostana* fruit rind extract. Bangkok: Mahidol University; 2009.
[47] Ong ES. Extraction methods and chemical standardization of botanicals and herbal preparations. *J. Chromatogr. B. Analyt. Technol. Biomed. Life Sci.* 2004 Dec 5;812(1-2):23-33.
[48] Pothitirat W, Chomnawang MT, Supabphol R, Gritsanapan W. Free radical scavenging and anti-acne activities of mangosteen fruit rind extracts prepared by different extraction methods. *Pharm. Biol.* 2010 Feb;48(2):182-6.
[49] Pothitirat W, Chomnawang MT, Gritsanapan W. Anti-acne inducing bacteria activity and alpha-mangostin content of *Garcinia mangostana* fruit rind extracts from different provenience. *Songklanakarin J. Sci. Technol.* 2008;31(1):41-7.
[50] Pothitirat W, Pithayanukul P, Chomnawang MT, Supabphol R, Gritsanapan W. Biological and chemical stability of mangosteen fruit rind extract. *Functional Plant Science and Biotechnology.* 2009;3(1):16-8.
[51] Pothitirat W, Gritsanapan W. Thin-layer chromatography-densitometric analysis of alpha-mangostin content in Garcinia mangostana fruit rind extracts. *J. AOAC Int.* 2008 Sep-Oct;91(5):1145-8.

[52] Pothitirat W, Gritsanapan W. HPLC quantitative analysis method for the determination of alpha-mangostin in mangosteen fruit rind extract. *Thai Journal of Agricultural Science.* 2009;42(1):7-12.

[53] Pothitirat W, Chomnawang MT, Supabphol R, Gritsanapan W. Comparison of bioactive compounds content, free radical scavenging and anti-acne inducing bacteria activities of extracts from the mangosteen fruit rind at two stages of maturity. *Fitoterapia.* 2009 Oct;80(7):442-7.

[54] Suksamrarn S, Suwannapoch N, Phakhodee W, Thanuhiranlert J, Ratananukul P, Chimnoi N, et al. Antimycobacterial activity of prenylated xanthones from the fruits of Garcinia mangostana. *Chem. Pharm. Bull.* (Tokyo). 2003 Jul;51(7):857-9.

[55] Chanarat P, Chanarat N, Fujihara M, Nagumo T. Immunopharmacological activity of polysaccharide from the pericarb of mangosteen garcinia: phagocytic intracellular killing activities. *J. Med. Assoc. Thai.* 1997 Sep;80 Suppl 1:S149-54.

[56] Iinuma M, Tosa H, Tanaka T, Asai F, Kobayashi Y, Shimano R, et al. Antibacterial activity of xanthones from guttiferaeous plants against methicillin-resistant Staphylococcus aureus. *J. Pharm. Pharmacol.* 1996 Aug;48(8):861-5.

[57] Sakagami Y, Iinuma M, Piyasena KG, Dharmaratne HR. Antibacterial activity of alpha-mangostin against vancomycin resistant Enterococci (VRE) and synergism with antibiotics. *Phytomedicine.* 2005 Mar;12(3):203-8.

[58] Voravuthikunchai SP, Kitpipit L. Activity of medicinal plant extracts against hospital isolates of methicillin-resistant Staphylococcus aureus. *Clin. Microbiol. Infect.* 2005 Jun; 11(6):510-2.

[59] Chomnawang MT, Surassmo S, Nukoolkarn VS, Gritsanapan W. Effect of Garcinia mangostana on inflammation caused by Propionibacterium acnes. *Fitoterapia.* 2007 Sep;78(6):401-8.

[60] Chin YW, Jung HA, Chai H, Keller WJ, Kinghorn AD. Xanthones with quinone reductase-inducing activity from the fruits of Garcinia mangostana (Mangosteen). *Phytochemistry.* 2008 Feb;69(3):754-8.

[61] Devi Sampath P, Vijayaraghavan K. Cardioprotective effect of alpha-mangostin, a xanthone derivative from mangosteen on tissue defense system against isoproterenol-induced myocardial infarction in rats. *J. Biochem. Mol. Toxicol.* 2007;21(6):336-9.

[62] Sukma M, Tohda M, Suksamran S, Tantisira B. gamma-Mangostin increases serotonin 2A/2C, muscarinic, histamine and bradykinin

receptor mRNA expression. *J. Ethnopharmacol.* 2011 May 17;135(2):450-4.
[63] Bumrungpert A, Kalpravidh RW, Chitchumroonchokchai C, Chuang CC, West T, Kennedy A, et al. Xanthones from mangosteen prevent lipopolysaccharide-mediated inflammation and insulin resistance in primary cultures of human adipocytes. *J. Nutr.* 2009 Jun;139(6):1185-91.
[64] Chen LG, Yang LL, Wang CC. Anti-inflammatory activity of mangostins from Garcinia mangostana. *Food Chem. Toxicol.* 2008 Feb;46(2):688-93.
[65] Nabandith V, Suzui M, Morioka T, Kaneshiro T, Kinjo T, Matsumoto K, et al. Inhibitory effects of crude alpha-mangostin, a xanthone derivative, on two different categories of colon preneoplastic lesions induced by 1, 2-dimethylhydrazine in the rat. *Asian Pac. J. Cancer Prev.* 2004 Oct-Dec;5(4):433-8.
[66] Nakagawa Y, Iinuma M, Naoe T, Nozawa Y, Akao Y. Characterized mechanism of alpha-mangostin-induced cell death: caspase-independent apoptosis with release of endonuclease-G from mitochondria and increased miR-143 expression in human colorectal cancer DLD-1 cells. *Bioorg. Med. Chem.* 2007 Aug 15;15(16):5620-8.
[67] Moongkarndi P, Kosem N, Kaslungka S, Luanratana O, Pongpan N, Neungton N. Antiproliferation, antioxidation and induction of apoptosis by Garcinia mangostana (mangosteen) on SKBR3 human breast cancer cell line. *J. Ethnopharmacol.* 2004 Jan;90(1):161-6.
[68] Balunas MJ, Su B, Brueggemeier RW, Kinghorn AD. Natural products as aromatase inhibitors. *Anticancer Agents Med. Chem.* 2008 Aug;8(6):646-82.
[69] Matsumoto K, Akao Y, Kobayashi E, Ohguchi K, Ito T, Tanaka T, et al. Induction of apoptosis by xanthones from mangosteen in human leukemia cell lines. *J. Nat. Prod.* 2003 Aug;66(8):1124-7.
[70] Matsumoto K, Akao Y, Yi H, Ohguchi K, Ito T, Tanaka T, et al. Preferential target is mitochondria in alpha-mangostin-induced apoptosis in human leukemia HL60 cells. *Bioorg. Med. Chem.* 2004 Nov 15;12(22):5799-806.
[71] Ho CK, Huang YL, Chen CC. Garcinone E, a xanthone derivative, has potent cytotoxic effect against hepatocellular carcinoma cell lines. *Planta Med.* 2002 Nov;68(11):975-9.

[72] Ee GC, Daud S, Izzaddin SA, Rahmani M. Garcinia mangostana: a source of potential anti-cancer lead compounds against CEM-SS cell line. *J. Asian Nat. Prod. Res*. 2008 May-Jun;10(5-6):475-9.

In: Acne
Editor: Mohamed L. Elsaie

ISBN: 978-1-62618-358-2
© 2013 Nova Science Publishers, Inc.

Chapter IV

Acne and IGF-I: A Fascinating Hypothesis

Elena Guanziroli, Laura Maffeis and Mauro Barbareschi
Department of Anaesthesiology,
Intensive Care and Dermatological Sciences,
Università degli Studi di Milano, Fondazione IRCCS,
Ca' Granda Ospedale Maggiore Policlinico, Milan, Italy

Abstract

Acne vulgaris is a common chronic inflammatory disease that affects the pilosebaceous follicle. Its pathophysiology is complex and multifactorial, with strong evidence supporting the involvement of increased sebum production, abnormal differentiation of skin keratinocytes, bacterial colonization, and inflammation. Recent experimental studies have suggested that acne is influenced by insulin/ insulin-like growth factor-1 (IGF-1) –signalling and may be considered an IGF-1-mediated disease. The purpose of this review article consists in delineating the role of insulin/ IGF-1 pathway in the pathogenesis of acne, its relationship with androgen hormones and the possible pharmacological and dietary intervention in restoring its equilibrium. The IGF-1 activity rises during puberty by the action of increased GH secretion and is amplified by insulin, which inhibits the production of

IGF binding protein-1 (IGFBP-1). Diets rich in carbohydrates with a high glycaemic index, which are associated with hyperglycaemia and reactive hyperinsulinaemia, increase formation of IGF-1. In addition to this, the *P. acnes*, which alone is able to activate the keratinocyte IGF-1/IGF-1 receptor system has also a central role in comedogenesis. IGF-1 promotes and maintains the expression of steroidogenic enzymes that are responsible for converting cholesterol into steroid precursors for the synthesis of dehydroepiandrosterone (DHEA) and androgens. Steroidogenic enzymes are expressed in human sebaceous glands where they may stimulate local androgen production. Moreover, IGF-1 can induce 5alpha-reductase in human skin fibroblasts, leading to an increased conversion of testosterone to dihydrotestosterone (DHT). It has recently been demonstrated that IGF-1 can increase lipid production in sebocytes *in vitro* via the activation of IGF-1 receptor through multiple pathways. Clinically, significantly higher IGF-1 levels have been described in women with acne compared with control subjects. The number of total acne lesions, inflammatory lesions, and serum levels of DHT are related with serum IGF-1 levels in women with acne. A correlation between the mean facial sebum excretion rate and serum IGF-1 levels has been shown in postadolescent acne patients. Pharmacological down-regulation of insulin/ IGF-1 signaling has been demonstrated with metformin, oral isotretinoin, and zinc treatment. These are promising options for the treatment of acne vulgaris, and conditions with insulin resistence, and increased IGF-1 serum levels. Patients with persistent acne, and with endocrine disorders, especially those with genetic variations of the IGF1 gene expressing increased IGF-1 serum levels, may benefit from dietary modifications including a reduction of dairy and hyperglycaemic foods.

The Insulin/IGF-1 Signaling

Growth hormone (GH) or somatotropin is a peptide produced by the pituitary gland. Its secretion is stimulated by hypothalamic GH-releasing hormone and inhibited by somatostatin, another peptide hormone secreted from the hypothalamus [1].

It is an important factor for organ growth and cell differentiation [2] and has a direct action through binding to the GH receptor (GHR) [3].

Activation of GHR induces the synthesis of IGF-1 protein in most tissues, with the liver being the organ that contributes the major part to serum IGF-1 level [4].

Since GH is released in intermittent secretory bursts and is thus impractical to asses by random serum sampling, increased levels have not been directly demonstrated in patients with acne. On the other hand, IGF-1 is relatively stable and primarily reflects cumulative secretion of GH, which makes it more suitable for serum testing. IGF-1 is a family of GH-dependent polypeptides homologous to insulin which stimulate in vivo and in vitro cell proliferation. IGF-1 has been localized in the peripheral cells of sebaceous glands in the rat [5]. In human skin appendages, the strongest expression of IGF-1 protein was found in maturing sebocytes and suprabasal cells of sebaceous ducts [6]. Endocrine and paracrine functions of IGF-I are modulated by a system of six circulating binding proteins (IGFBP 1–6) and their proteases [7]. In the circulation, about 75% of IGF-I is bound to IGFBP-3, but the primary and unique regulator of IGF-I bioavailability in response to changes in the circulating insulin levels appears to be IGFBP-1 [8]. IGFBP-1 promoter region contains the insulin response element (IRE) and insulin appears to be the primary determinant of IGFBP-1 expression via its inhibition of IGFBP-1 transcription [9]. The IGF1R is a tyrosine kinase receptor, which is able to form heterodimers with insulin receptor (IR) [1].

Insulin may act as an IGF-I surrogate as it has approximately 50% amino acid homology to the insulin-like growth factors (IGFs), and it binds to the IGF-I receptor at high concentrations with an affinity 100-fold less than to its native receptor [10]. Circulating IGF-I levels are often used as a substitute for tissue IGF-I bioactivity due to the lack of *in vivo* methods to measure bioactivity. The majority of the circulating IGF-I levels come from the liver, but IGF bioactivity in tissues is related not only to circulating IGF and IGF-binding protein levels, but also genetic and local production [11]. Despite the number of factors such as multiple hormones, nutrition, age and sex that may influence IGF-I levels, it has been estimated that up to 60% of the variability has a genetic basis [11].

Role of IGF-1 in the Pathogenesis of Acne Vulgaris

Correlation between Acne and Insulin/IGF-1 Signaling

Acne vulgaris is a common chronic inflammatory skin disease of the pilosebaceous unit, affecting more than 85% of adolescents. It is seen in nearly

100% of individuals at some time during their lives [12]. For some, it is temporary and resolves by the mid-20s; however, more severe cases often take longer to resolve, and can persist into adult years [13].

It is characterized by both inflammatory (papules, pustules, nodules) and noninflammatory (comedones, open and closed) lesions, less frequently by nodules, or pseudocysts and, in some cases, it is accompanied by scarring [14].

The main pathophysiologic factors influencing the development of acne are: sebaceous gland hyperplasia with seborrhea, pilosebaceous unit obstruction by abnormal keratinization, Propionibacterium acnes colonization of the follicle and inflammation mediated by both chemotactic factors and various enzymes.

Several hormones implicated in the regulation of sebaceous gland activity have been linked to acne. They include androgens, estrogens, progesterone, adrenocorticotropic hormone (ACTH), glucocorticoids, GH, and IGF-1 [15].

A growing body of evidence underlines the role of insulin resistance with increased insulin/IGF-1 signalling in the pathogenesis of acne.

Expression of acne during adolescence is associated with endocrine variations, which are closely related to changes in insulin sensitivity. In fact, during normal puberty and adolescence, there is a transient decline in insulin sensitivity [16, 17], which is accompanied by a reciprocal decrease in levels of SHBG and IGFBP-1 [18]. According to cross-sectional observations, acne begins about the same time as the gradual increase in plasma insulin [16], the preadolescent increase in body mass index (BMI) [19], and the increase in IGF-I concentrations [16, 17]. Acne incidence corresponds less closely to plasma androgen levels than it does to insulin and IGF-I levels [20, 21]. This is because insulin and IGF-I levels peak during late puberty and gradually decline until the third decade [16]. Acne generally resolves by this time despite circulating androgens remain unchanged.

Recent studies describe a correlation between IGF-1 serum levels and the severity of acne in women [22, 23].

Individuals with Laron syndrome who carry mutations in the growth hormone receptor (GHR) gene that lead to severe congenital IGF-1 deficiency with decreased insulin/IGF-1 signaling exhibit reduced prevalence rates of acne, diabetes and cancer [24].

Moreover, IGF-I (CA) 19 polymorphism was statistically different in acne patients compared with healthy controls and it may be associated with acne severity [25].

The Insulin/IGF-1 Signaling and Sebaceous Lipogenesis

Sebaceous glands are found all over the human body, with the exception of the palms and soles, and are most numerous on the scalp and the face. The embryologic development of the human sebaceous gland is closely related to the differentiation of the hair follicle and the epidermis [26]. Together with the hair follicles, they comprise the pilosebaceous unit [27]. The number of sebaceous glands remains approximately the same throughout life, whereas their size tends to increase with age. The development and function of the sebaceous gland in the fetal and neonatal periods appear to be regulated by maternal androgens and by endogenous steroid synthesis. The most apparent function of the glands is to excrete sebum. Patients with acne have larger sebaceous glands and produce more sebum than do those without acne [26].

GH and IGF-1 may play roles in sebaceous gland physiology as evidenced by the expression of receptors of GH and IGF-1 on human sebaceous glands and in sebocytes [28].

In hypophysectomized rat experiments, GH increased sebum excretion, acting synergically with testostetone (T) [29].

The rate of sebum excretion has been shown to be abnormally high in patients with acromegaly [30].

Other reports indicate that GH may act directly on the sebaceous glands via a GH receptor/binding protein [31, 32].

A role for IGF-1 and insulin in stimulating sebaceous gland lipogenesis was first demonstrated in rat preputial sebocytes [33].

Lipogenesis is also stimulated by IGF-1 in sebaceous glands grown in organ culture [34].

Furthermore, studies show that IGF-1 increases lipogenesis in the SEB-1 sebocyte model inducing an increase in expression of sterol response element binding protein-1 (SREBP-1).

The sterol response element-binding proteins (SREBPs) are nuclear transcription factors that regulate the synthesis of numerous genes involved in lipid biosynthesis. As suggested by their name, SREBPs bind sterol response elements in the promoters of genes involved in lipogenesis, including fatty acid synthase, long-chain fatty acyl elongase, stearoyl CoA desaturase, HMG CoA synthase, HMG CoA reductase, and squalene synthase [35].

SREBP-1c increases also in response to insulin signalling [36]. SREBP-1 has been implicated in the development of insulin resistance and regulates components of the insulin signalling pathway such as IRS-2 and PI3KR3 [37].

IGF-1 serum levels also correlate directly with the amount of facial sebum in both men and women [38].

The IGF-1/IGF-1R System and P. Acnes

Propionibacterium acnes (P.acnes) proliferates in the lipid-rich sebaceous follicles and induces an inflammatory reaction but also maintains it. It secretes chemotactic factors and increases the secretion of proinflammatory cytokines (tumor necrosis factor-α, IL-1β, and IL-8), from mononuclear cells and keratinocytes [39, 40].

P. acnes also induces the activation of Toll-like receptors-2 and -4 in keratinocytes [41].

Furthermore, the *P. acnes* genome encodes many factors that may have inflammatory potential [42].

In addition, it produces a number of extracellular enzymes and metabolites that can directly damage host tissue.

One of the well-known enzymes is the extracellular triacylglycerol lipase that produces free fatty acids (FFAs) by hydrolyzing triglycerides in sebum.

Sebum FFAs, if overproduced, induce very mild inflammation and promote bacterial adherence and colonization in sebaceous follicles [43].

It was recently reported that P.acnes alone stimulates IGF-1 and IGF-1R expression in keratinocytes and increases IGF-1 secretion [44].

Moreover, IGF-1 and IGF-1R overexpression in both acne lesions and skin explants is associated with an increase in Ki-67 and filaggrin expression in the epidermis, confirming that the IGF-1/IGF-1R system is associated with the modulation of both proliferation and differentiation of keratinocytes [44].

The Insulin/IGF-1 Signaling and Androgen

The development of acne is dependent on the presence of IGF-1 and the close interrelationship of IGF-1 with androgens.

Androgens are major regulators of sebaceous gland function.

Human sebaceous glands can produce testosterone by *de novo* synthesis from abundant serum cholesterol and via a shortcut pathway by using circulating DHEA and possibly other circulating testosterone precursors [45].

The importance of androgens in sebaceous gland function is well recognized. Studies have shown that women with acne have significantly higher levels of plasma androgen (although still within normal range) than women without acne [46], and that the concentration of dehydroepiandrosterone sulphate (DHEA-S) is significantly and specifically associated with the initiation of acne in young girls [47].

Increasing levels of serum androgens appear to correlate with a rise in IGF-1 level.

A significant positive correlation between serum DHEAS and serum IGF-1 was found in prepubertal girls, indicating that GH/IGF axis might be an important metabolic signal involved in the maturational change of human adrenal androgens during prepuberty [48].

In a recent study DHT correlated with serum IGF-1 in women with clinical acne, while DHEAS and androstenedione levels correlated with IGF-1 in affected men [23].

Similarly, when oophorectomized women were given testosterone (T), a linear increase occurred in the IGF-1-IGFBP-3 ratio [49].

T has been reported to stimulate IGF-1 levels in prepubertal males with sufficient acne secretion [50].

The administration of recombinant IGF-1 in patients with Laron syndrome was associated with a progressive rise in LH and testosterone in both male and female patients [51].

Effects of the Insulin/IGF-1 Signaling on the Adrenal Gland, Gonads, 5α-Reductase and Androgen Receptor

The GH-IGF-1 axis plays an important role for the ACTH-dependent production of DHEAS of the human adrenal gland [52, 53]. IGF-1 enhances the sensitivity of the adrenal for ACTH, and induces the expression and activity of key enzymes of adrenal androgen biosynthesis [53].

IGF-1 stimulates the estrogen synthesis by granulosa cells [54] and both IGF-1 and IGF-2 enhance the efficacy of luteinizing hormone (LH) stimulation of interstitial theca-cells, increasing ovarian androgen production [55], suggesting that the IGF-system may play a role in the pathogenesis of ovarian hyperandrogenism and polycystic ovary syndrome (PCOS) [55].

The IGF system is important for Leydig cell differentiation, mitogenesis, antiapoptosis, and androgen biosynthesis in the testes [56, 57, 58].

Adult Leydig cells are responsible for increasing the circulating levels of pubertal androgens [59]. IGF-1 messenger RNA, IGF-1 protein, and IGF1R have been identified in Leydig cells, peritubular cells, and spermatocytes [56, 57]. In addition, inhibition of IGF1R, resulting in less IGF-1 locally, increases Leydig cell apoptosis [58].

IGF-1 and LH together stimulate proliferation of Leydig-cell precursors, and IGF-1 is an essential local mediator of DNA synthesis and steroidogenesis [59].Testicular IGF-1 levels increase during puberty in conjunction with an increase of testosterone production. In rat and human scrotal skin fibroblasts, IGF-1 increases 5α-reductase activity, suggesting that IGF-1 has a role as a peripheral amplifier of androgen metabolism in the skin [60].

IGF-1 induces androgen receptor (AR) trans-activation. In the nucleus, AR binds to the AR repressive protein Foxo1. IGF-1, as well as insulin activates PI3K, which leads to Akt-mediated Foxo1 phosphorylation. Phosphorylated Foxo1 leaves the AR and translocates from the nucleus into the cytoplasm [61]. By this mechanism, IGF-1 signalling alleviates AR repression resulting in AR gain-of-function.

Thus, IGF-1 has direct influence on the intracrine androgen regulation of the skin and potentiates androgen signalling by the induction of 5α-reductase activity and activation of AR.

Insulin has been shown to stimulate ovarian androgen production through effects on steroidogenic enzymes and by amplifying gonadotrophin-releasing hormone secretion [62]. Insulin stimulates adrenal androgen synthesis [63] and inhibit hepatic SHBG production [64] in the liver resulting in increased concentrations of free testosterone.

Clinical and experimental evidence suggests that insulin resistance and its compensatory hyperinsulinemia are the underlying disturbance in PCOS, as insulin resistance generally precedes and gives rise to hyperandrogenism [65].

The Insulin/IGF-1 Signaling in the Transcriptional Regulation

There is indirect evidence supporting the role of GH/IGF-1 axis in posttranslational modification of nuclear FoxO1 and strengthens the hypothesis of a nuclear FoxO1 deficiency as the possible underlying cause of acne and clinical acne variants.

FoxO1 has been identified as an important regulatory protein of that modulates the expression of genes involved in cell cycle control, DNA damage repair, apoptosis, androgen receptor, cell differentiation, apoptosis, oxidative stress regulation, innate and acquired immunity. Nuclear FoxO1 down regulation is the result of increased insulin/IGF-1 signaling with the consequent activation of phosphoinositol-3-kinase (PI3K) and Akt kinase. Reduced nuclear levels of FoxO1 may increase the expression of important acne target genes and derepress nuclear receptors involved in the clinical manifestation of acne [66].

The Insulin/IGF-1 Signaling and Diet

Historically, the relationship between diet and acne has been highly controversial.

Many previous reports have shown no relationship between food and acne [67-71]. However, cumulating evidence supports the view that the typical Western diet, consisting of numerous dairy sources and foods with high glycemic indices, produces hyperglycemia, reactive hyperinsulinemia, and increased formation of IGF-1 [72].

An association between acne and mild peripheral insulin resistance has been previously described in healthy eumenorrheic women [73].

Accumulating evidence suggests that low glycemic–load (LGL) diets may play a dual role in the prevention of hyperinsulinemia by lowering the postprandial insulin demand and improving insulin sensitivity [74, 75].

Cordain et al. recently proposed that a high glycemic load Western diet may frequently expose adolescents to significant hyperinsulinemia and a hormonal cascade that favors increased keratinocyte growth and sebum production [76].

Diets with a low glycaemic load decreased serum IGF-1 levels and significantly improved acne following a 12-week diet [77]. The endocrine effects of low glycaemic load versus a high glycaemic load diet on 12 male acne patients showed a significant increase in IGFBP-1 and IGFBP-3 in the low glycaemic load group, suggesting that low glycaemic diet reduces free IGF-1 activity and bioavailablity [78].

Milk contains carbohydrates, including of course lactose, and its consumption produces a glycemic response and an insulinemic response.

The insulinemic response to ingested milk is actually three to six times what would be expected or predicted from the carbohydrate load in the milk serving [79].This is true for skimmed and full-fat milk, but not for cheese [80, 81].

High milk consumption increases IGF-1 levels 10% to 20% in adults and 20% to 30% in children [82-84], and milk and dairy products raise IGF-1 levels more than dietary protein such as meat [84].

In 2109 European women, serum IGF-1 levels were positively related with the intake of milk [85].

Prolonged consumption of ultraheat-treated (UHT) milk shifts the GH/IGF-1 axis in children to higher levels [86].

After a month of drinking 710 ml of UHT milk daily, Mongolian children, who had not previously consumed milk, had a higher mean plasma level of IGF-1, higher IGF-1/IGFBP-3 and GH levels [86].

Their mean serum IGF-1 levels were significantly raised after 4 weeks of milk consumption by 23.4% [86].

Prospective cohort studies in the United States in 4273 teenage boys and 6094 teenage girls demonstrated a correlation between milk consumption and acne [87, 88]. In boys, the strongest association has been found between intake of skim milk and acne [88]. Skim milk has been identified as a potent insulin secretagogue in type 2 diabetic patients [89].

Thus, it is conceivable that not the lipophilic androgenic steroids enriched in milk fat [90], but more likely the hydrophilic protein fraction in cow's milk, which increases insulin/IGF-1 signalling, might have a stronger influence on the milk-induced aggravation of acne.

Some of the most compelling evidence suggesting an association between diet and acne comes from patients with polycystic ovarian syndrome, a condition with a constellation of features including insulin resistance, hyperinsulinemia, hyperandrogenism, and acne [91]. Studies have demonstrated that acne improves when these patients are treated with medications that improve insulin metabolism such as metformin, tolbutamide, pioglitazone, and acarbose [92, 93].

Treatments of Acne Which Modulate Insulin/IGF-1 Signaling

Isotretinoin (13-cis retinoic acid), metformin, acarbose and zinc gluconate may have a negative influence on the insulin/IGF-1 axis.

The influence of isotretinoin on GH physiology was suggested by a significant decrease in IGF-1 and IGFBP3 levels after 3 months of treatment [94].

A recent review demonstrated that oral isotretinoin treatment acts on all major pathogenetic factors of acne by restoring the FoxO activity, which is the most important target of retinoids action [66].

The use of insulin-sensitizing agents improving insulin resistance provided a new option in the treatment of hyperinsulinemic PCOS women. Metformin is a biguanide used in treatment of type 2 diabetes; this agent inhibits hepatic glucose synthesis, intestinal glucose absorption, and increases insulin sensitivity in the peripheral tissues, but does not cause hypoglycemia [95].

Metformin therapy not only normalizes levels of insulin and testosterone, but also decreases the pool of free-bioactive IGF-I by increasing the levels of circulating IGFBP-1 in women with polycystic ovary syndrome [96].

In PCOS patients, metformin as well as rosiglitazone significantly increased GLUT4 mRNA expression, leading to an increased uptake of glucose [97].

Acarbose, an α-glucosidase inhibitor, has been shown able to flatten the post-prandial glucose and insulin increase and to decrease the serum androgen concentrations in hyperinsulinaemic pre-menopausal women with hypertestosteronaema [98].

Ciotta et al. recently demonstrated a 46% reduction of the acne/seborrehea score in PCOS women treated with acarbose.

The clinical improvement was associated with a significant reduction in the insulin response to an oral glucose load, a decreasing in androgen concentrations, with a significant rise in SHBG levels [93].

Zinc salts have demonstrated their efficacy in inflammatory acne treatment as well as their bacteriostatic activity against Propionibacterium acnes [99].

A link between zinc and the IGF-1 system has been reported in the downregulation of IGF-1R expression in prostate cancer cells [100].

Very recently, it has been shown that zinc gluconate had the effect of downregulating IGF-1 and IGF-1R levels [101].

References

[1] Edmondson SR, Thumiger SP, Werther GA, Wraight CJ. Epidermal homeostasis: the role of growth hormone and insulin-like growth factor systems. *Endocr. Rev.* 2003; 24(6):737-764.

[2] Nixon BT, Green H. Growth hormone promotes the differentiation of myoblasts and preadipocytes generated by azacytidine treatment of 10T 1/2 cells. *Proc. Natl. Acad. Sci. USA.* 1984; 81(11):3429-3432.
[3] Green H, Morikawa M, Nixon T. A dual effector theory of growth-hormone action. *Differentiation.* 1985;29(3):195-198.
[4] Isaksson OG, Lindahl A, Nilsson A, Isgaard J. Mechanism of the stimulatory effect of growth hormone on longitudinal bone growth. *Endocr. Rev.* 1987;8(4):426-438.
[5] Hansson HA, Nilsson A, Isgaard J et al. Immunohistochemical localization of insulin-like growth factor-I in the adult rat. *Histochemistry.* 1988;89(4):403-410.
[6] Rudman SM, Philpott MP, Thomas GA, Kealey T. The role of IGF-I in human skin and its appendages: morphogen as well as mitogen? *J. Invest. Dermatol.* 1997;109(6):770-777.
[7] Poretsky L, Cataldo N, Rosenwaks Z, Giudice L. The insulin-related ovarian regulatory system in health and disease. *Endocr. Rev.* 1999;20(4):535-582.
[8] Baxter R. Insulin-like growth factor binding proteins in the human circulation: a review. *Horm. Res.* 1994;42(4-5):140-144.
[9] Lee P, Giudice L, Conover C, Powel D. Insulin-like growth factor binding protein-1: recent findings and new directions. *Proc. Soc. Exp. Biol. Med.* 1997;216(3):319-357.
[10] Jones JI, Clemmons DR. Insulin-like growth factors and their binding proteins: biological actions. *Endocr. Rev.* 1995;16(1):3-34.
[11] Cleveland RJ, Gammon MD, Edmiston SN et al. IGF1 CA repeat polymorphisms, lifestyle factors and breast cancer risk in the Long Island Breast Cancer Study Project. *Carcinogenesis.* 2006;27(4):758-765.
[12] Sandra LH, Davidson S, Smith CB. Cause and effect: the relationship between acne and self-esteem in adolescent years. *J. Nurs. Pract.* 2008;4:595-600.
[13] Thiboutot D, Gollnick H, Bettoli V, et al. New insights into the management of acne: an update from the global alliance to improve outcomes in acne group. *J. Am. Acad. Dermatol.* 2009;60(5)(Supp 5):S1-S50.
[14] Burns T, Breathnach S, Cox N, Griffith C. *Rook's textbook of dermatology.* 7th ed. Massachusetts, USA: Blackwell Publishing Company; 2004;43.1–43.78.

[15] Melnik BC, Schmitz G. Role of insulin, insulin-like growth factor-1, hyperglycaemic food and milk consumption in the pathogenesis of acne vulgaris. *Exp. Dermatol.* 2009;1(10):1-9.

[16] Smith C, Dunger D, AJK W, et al. Relationship between insulin, insulin-like growth factor I, and dehydroepiandrosterone sulfate concentrations during childhood, puberty and adult life. *J. Clin. Endocrinol. Metab.* 1989;68(5):932-937.

[17] Caprio S, Plewe G, Diamond M, al. Increased insulin secretion in puberty: a compensatory response to reductions in insulin sensitivity. *J. Pediatr.* 1989;114(6):963-967.

[18] Holly J, Smith C, Dunger D, et al. Relationship between the pubertal fall in sex hormone binding globulin and insulin-like growth factor binding protein-I: a synchronized approach to pubertal development? *Clin. Endocrinol.* 1989;31(3):277-284.

[19] Rolland-Cachera M. Body composition during adolescence: methods, limitations and determinants. *Horm. Res.* 1993;39(Suppl 3):25–40.

[20] Cara JF, Rosenfield RL, Furlanetto RW. A longitudinal study of the relationship of plasma somatomedin-C concentration to the pubertal growth spurt. *Am. J. Dis. Child.* 1987;141(5):562–564.

[21] Albertsson-Wikland K, Rosberg S, Karlberg J, Groth T. Analysis of 24-hour growth hormone profiles in healthy boys and girls of normal stature: relation to puberty. *J. Clin. Endocrinol. Metab.* 1994;78(5):1195–1201.

[22] Aizawa H, Niimura M. Elevated serum insulin-like growth factor-1 (IGF-1) levels in women with postadolescent acne. *J. Dermatol.* 1995;22(4):249-252.

[23] Cappel M, Mauger D, Thiboutot D. Correlation between serum levels of insulin-like growth factor 1, dehydroepiandrosterone sulfate, and dihydrotestosterone and acne lesion counts in adult women. *Arch. Dermatol.* 2005;141(3):333-338.

[24] Melnik BC, John SM, Schmitz G. Over-stimulation of insulin/IGF-1 signaling by western diet may promote diseases of civilization: lessons learnt from laron syndrome. *Nutr. Metab.* 2011;24(8):41.

[25] Tasli L, Turgut S, Kacar N, et al. Insulin-like growth factor-I gene polymorphism in acne vulgaris. *J. Eur. Acad. Dermatol. Venereol.* 2011. doi: 10.1111/j.1468-3083.2011. 04299.

[26] Zouboulis C. Acne and sebaceous gland function. *Clin. Dermatol.* 2004;22(5):360-366.

[27] Lucky AW. Quantitative documentation of a premenstrual flare of facial acne in adult women. *Arch. Dermatol.* 2004;140(4):423-424.
[28] Rudman SM, Philpott MP, Thomas GA, Kealey T. The role of IGF-I in human skin and its appendages: morphogen as well as mitogen?_*J. Invest. Dermatol.* 1997;109(6):770-777.
[29] Ebling FJ, Ebling E, Randall V, Skinner J. The sebotrophic action of growth hormone (BGH) in the rat._*Br. J. Dermatol.* 1975;92(3):325-332.
[30] Burton JL, Libman LJ, Cunliffe WJ, et al. Sebum excretion in acromegaly. *Br. Med. J.* 1972;1(5797):406-408.
[31] Lobie PE, Breipohl W, Lincoln DT, García-Aragón J, Waters MJ. Localization of the growth hormone receptor/binding protein in skin. *J. Endocrinol.* 1990;126(3):467-471.
[32] Oakes SR, Haynes KM, Waters MJ, Herington AC, Werther GA. Demonstration and localization of growth hormone receptor in human skin and skin fibroblasts._*J. Clin. Endocrinol. Metab.* 1992;75(5):1368-1373.
[33] Deplewski D, Rosenfield RL. Growth hormone and insulin-like growth factors have different effects on sebaceous cell growth and differentiation. *Endocrinology.* 1999;140(9):4089-4094.
[34] Downie MM, Guy R, Kealey T.Advances in sebaceous gland research: potential new approaches to acne management. *Int. J. Cosmetic Sci.* 2004;26(6):291-311.
[35] Horton JD. Sterol regulatory element-binding proteins: transcriptional activators of lipid synthesis. *Biochem. Soc. Trans.* 2002;30(6):1091-1095.
[36] Foretz M, Guichard C, Ferré P, Foufelle F. Sterol regulatory element binding protein-1c is a major mediator of insulin action on the hepatic expression of glucokinase and lipogenesis-related genes. *Proc. Natl. Acad. Sci. USA.* 1999;96(22):12737-12742.
[37] Kallin A, Johannessen L E, Cani P D et al. SREBP-1 regulates the expression of heme oxygenase I and the phosphatidylinositol-3 kinase regulatory subunit p55gamma. *J. Lipid Res.* 2007;48(7):1628-1636.
[38] Vora S, Ovhal A, Jerajani H et al. Correlation of facial sebum to serum insulin-like growth factor-1 in patients with acne. *Br. J. Dermatol.* 2008;159(7):990-991.
[39] Vowels BR, Yang S, Leyden JJ. Induction of proinflammatory cytokines by a soluble factor of Propionibacterium acnes: implications for chronic inflammatory acne. *Infect. Immun.* 1995;63(8):3158-3165.

[40] Sugisaki H, Yamanaka K, Kakeda M et al. Increased interferon-gamma, interleukin-12p40 and IL-8 production in Propionibacterium acnes–treated peripheral blood mononuclear cells from patient with acne vulgaris: host response but not bacterial species is the determinant factor of the disease. *J. Dermatol. Sci.* 2009;55(1):47-52.

[41] Jugeau S, Tenaud I, Knol AC et al. Induction of toll-like receptors by Propionibacterium acnes. *Br. J. Dermatol.* 2005;153(6):1105-1113.

[42] Bruggemann H, Henne A, Hoster F et al. The complete genome sequence of Propionibacterium acnes, a commensal of human skin. *Science.* 2004;305(5684): 671-673.

[43] Puhvel SM, Sakamoto M. A reevaluation of fatty acids as inflammatory agents in acne. *J. Invest. Dermatol.* 1977;68(2):93-97.

[44] Isard O, Knol AC, Ariès MF, et al. Propionibacterium acnes activates the IGF-1/IGF-1R system in the epidermis and induces keratinocyte proliferation. *J. Invest. Dermatol.* 2011;131(1):59-66.

[45] Chen W, Tsai SJ, Sheu HM, Tsai JC, Zouboulis CC. Testosterone synthesized in cultured human SZ95 sebocytes derives mainly from dehydroepiandrosterone. *Exp. Dermatol.* 2010;19(5):470-472.

[46] Thiboutot D, Gilliland K, Light J, Lookingbill D. Androgen metabolism in sebaceous glands from subjects with and without acne. *Arch. Dermatol.* 1999;135(5684): 1041-1045.

[47] Lucky AW, Biro FM, Huster GA, Leach AD, Morrison JA, Ratterman J. Acne vulgaris in premenarchal girls. An early sign of puberty associated with rising levels of dehydroepiandrosterone. *Arch. Dermatol.* 1994;130(3):308-314.

[48] Guercio G, Rivarola MA, Chaler E, Maceiras M, Belgorosky A. Relationship between the growth hormone/insulin-like growth factor-I axis, insulin sensitivity, and adrenal androgens in normal prepubertal and pubertal girls. *J. Clin. Endocrinol. Metab.* 2003;88(3): 1389-1393.

[49] Azziz R, Deal CL, Potter HD, Gargosky SE, Rosenfeld RG. Regulation of extragonadal insulin-like growth factor-binding protein-3 by testosterone in oophorectomized women. *J. Clin. Endocrinol. Metab.* 1994;79(6):1747-1751.

[50] Rosenfield RL, Furlanetto R. Physiologic testosterone or estradiol induction of puberty increases plasma somatomedin-C. *J. Pediatr.* 1985;107(3):415-417.

[51] Ben-Amitai D, Laron Z. Effect of insulin-like growth factor-1 deficiency or administration on the occurrence of acne. *J. Eur. Acad. Dermatol. Venereol.* 2011; 25(8):950-954.

[52] Belgorosky A, Baquedano M S, Guerico G, Rivarola M A. Adrenarche: postnatal adrenal zonation and hormonal and metabolic regulation. *Horm. Res.* 2008;70(5):257-267.
[53] Mesiano S, Katz S L, Lee J Y, Jaffe R B. Insulin-like growth factors augment steroid production and expression of steroidogeneic enzymes in human fetal adrenal cortical cells: implications for adrenal androgen regulation. *J. Clin. Endocrinol. Metabol.* 1997; 82(5):1390-1396.
[54] Giudice LC. Insulin-like growth factors and ovarian follicular development. *Endocr. Rev.* 1992;13(4):641-669.
[55] Cara JF. Insulin-like growth factors, insulin-like growth factor binding proteins and ovarian androgen production. *Horm. Res.* 1994;42(1-2):49-54.
[56] Berensztein EB, Baquedano MS, Pepe CM et al. Role of IGFs and insulin in the human testis during post natal activation: differentiation of steroidogenic cells. *Pediatr. Res.* 2008;63(6):662-666.
[57] Lin T, Wang DL, Calkins JH, Guo H, Chi R, Housley PR. Regulation of insulin-like growth factor-I messenger ribonucleic acid expression in Leydig cells. *Mol. Cell Endocrinol.* 1990;73(2-3):147-152.
[58] Colon E, Svechnikov KV, Carlsson-Skwirut C, Bang P, Soder O. Stimulation of steroidogenesis in immature rat Leydig cells evoked by interleukin-1alpha is potentiated by growth hormone and insulin-like growth factors. *Endocrinology.* 2005;146(1):221-230.
[59] Wang G, Hardy MP. Development of Leydig cells in the insulin-like growth factor-I (IGF-I) knockout mouse: effects of IGF-I replacement and gonadotropic stimulation. *Biol. Reprod.* 2004;70 (3):632-639.
[60] Horton R, Pasupuletti V, Antonipillai I. Androgen induction of steroid 5 alpha-reductase may be mediated via insulin-like growth factor-I. *Endocrinology.* 1993; 133(2):447-451.
[61] Fan W, Yanase T, Morinaga H et al. Insulin-like growth factor 1/insulin signaling activates androgen signaling through direct interactions of Foxo1 with androgen receptor. *J. Biol. Chem.* 2007: 282(10):7329-7338.
[62] Willis D, Mason H, Gilling-Smith C, Franks S. Modulation by insulin of follicle stimulating and luteinizing hormone action in human granulosa cells of normal and polycystic ovaries. *J. Clin. Endocrinol. Metab.* 1996;81(1):302-309.
[63] Kristiansen S, Endoh A, Casson P, Buster J, Hornsby P. Induction of steroidogenic enzyme genes by insulin and IGF-I in cultured adult human adrenocortical cells. *Steroids.* 1997;62(2):258-265.

[64] Singh A, Hamilton-Fairley D, Koistinen R, et al. Effect of insulin-like growth factor-type I (IGF-I) and insulin on the secretion of sex hormone binding globulin and IGF-I binding protein (IBP-I) by human hepatoma cells. *J. Endocrinol.* 1990;124(2):R1-3.
[65] Dunaif A, Segal K, Shelley D, Green G, Dorbrjansky A. Profound peripheral insulin resistance, independent of obesity in polycystic ovary syndrome. *Diabetes.* 1989; 38(9):1165-1174.
[66] Melnik BC. The role of transcription factor FoxO1 in the pathogenesis of acne vulgaris and the mode of isotretinoin action. *G Ital. Dermatol. Venereol.* 2010;145(5):559-571.
[67] Kaminester LH. Acne. *JAMA* 1978;239(20):2171-2172.
[68] Michaelsson G. Diet and acne. *Nutr. Rev.* 1981;39(2):104-106.
[69] Rasmussen JE. Diet and acne. *Int. J. Dermatol.* 1977;16(6):488-92.
[70] Loeffel ED. Foods and acne. *J. Tenn. Med. Assoc.* 1972;65(10):918.
[71] Bershad S. The unwelcome return of the acne diet. *Arch. Dermatol.* 2003;139(7):940-941.
[72] Melnik BC. Evidence for acne-promoting effects of milk and other insulinotropic dairy products. *Nestle Nutr. Workshop Ser. Pediatr. Program.* 2011;67:131-145.
[73] Aizawa H, Niimura M. Mild insulin resistance during oral glucose tolerance test (OGTT) in women with acne. *J. Dermatol.* 1996;23(8):526-529.
[74] Jenkins D, Kendall C, Augustin L et al. Glycemic index: overview of implications in healthy and disease. *Am. J. Clin. Nutr.* 2002;76(1):266S-273S.
[75] Carnethon MR, Loria CM, Hill JO, Sidney S, Savage PJ, Liu K. Risk factors for the metabolic syndrome: the coronary artery risk development in young adults (CARDIA) study, 1985-2001. *Diabetes Care.* 2004;27(11):2707-2715.
[76] Cordain L, Lindeberg S, Hurtado M., et al. Acne Vulgaris – A disease of Western civilization. *Arch. Dermatol.* 2002;138(12):1584-1590.
[77] Smith R, Mann N, Braue A, Mäkeläinen H, Varigos G A. The effect of a high protein, low glycemic load diet versus a conventional, high glycemic load diet on biochemical parameters associated with acne vulgaris. *J. Am. Acad. Dermatol.* 2007;57(2):247-256.
[78] Smith R, Mann N, Mäkeläinen H, Roper J, Braue A, Varigos G. A pilot study to determine the short-term effects of a low glycemic load diet on hormonal markers of acne: a nonrandomized, parallel, controlled feeding trial. *Mol. Nutr. Food Res.* 2008; 52(6):718-726.

[79] Ostman EM, Liljeberg Elmstahl HG, Bjorck IM. Inconsistency between glycemic and insulinemic responses to regular and fermented milk products. *Am. J. Clin. Nutr.* 2001; 74(1):96-100.
[80] Holt SH, Miller JC, Petocz P. An insulin index of foods: the insulin demand generated by 1000-kJ portions of common foods. *Am. J. Clin. Nutr.*1997;66(5):1264-1276.
[81] Hoyt G, Hickey MS, Cordain L. Dissociation of the glycaemic and insulinaemic responses to whole and skimmed milk. *Br. J. Nutr.* 2005;93(2):175-177.
[82] Hoppe C, Udam TR, Lauritzen L, Molgaard C, Juul A, Michaelsen KF. Animal protein intake, serum insulin-like growth factor I, and growth in healthy 2.5-y-old Danish children. *Am. J. Clin. Nutr.* 2004;80(2):447-452.
[83] Hoppe C, Molgaard C, Juul A, Michaelsen KF. High intakes of skimmed milk, but not meat, increase serum IGF-I and IGFBP-3 in eight-year-old boys. *Eur. J. Clin. Nutr.* 2004; 58(9):1211-1216.
[84] Hoppe C, Molgaard C, Vaag A, Barkholt V, Michaelsen KF. High intakes of milk, but not meat, increase s-insulin and insulin resistance in 8-year-old boys. *Eur. J. Clin. Nutr.* 2005;59(3):393-398.
[85] Norat T, Dossus L, Rinaldi S et al. Diet, serum insulin-like growth factor-I and IGF-binding protein-3 in European women. *Eur. J. Clin. Nutr.* 2007;61(1):91-98.
[86] Rich-Edwards JW, Ganmaa D, Pollak MN et al. Milk consumption and the prepubertal somatotropic axis. *Nutr. J.* 2007;6:28.
[87] Adebamowo CA, Spiegelman D, Berkey CS et al. Milk consumption and acne in adolescent girls. *Dermatol. Online J.* 2006; 12(4):1.
[88] Adebamowo CA, Spiegelman D, Berkey CS et al. Milk consumption and acne in teenaged boys. *J. Am. Acad. Dermatol.* 2008;58(5):787-793.
[89] Gannon MC, Nuttal FQ, Krezowski PA, Billington CJ, Parker S. The serum insulin and plasma glucose responses to milk and fruit in type 2 (non-insulin-dependent) diabetic patients. *Diabetologia.* 1986;29(11): 784-791.
[90] Danby FW. Acne, dairy and cancer. *Dermato-Endocrinology.* 2009;1(1):12-16.
[91] Marsh K, Brand-Miller J. The optimal diet for women with polycystic ovary syndrome? *Br. J. Nutr.* 2005;94(2):154-165.
[92] De Leo V, Musacchio MC, Morgante G, Piomboni P, Petraglia F. Metformin treatment is effective in obese teenage girls with PCOS. *Hum. Reprod.* 2006;21(9):2252-2256.

[93] Ciotta L, Calogero AE, Farina M, De Leo V, La Marca A, Cianci A. Clinical, endocrine and metabolic effects of acarbose, an alpha-glucosidase inhibitor, in PCOS patients with increased insulin response and normal glucose tolerance. *Hum. Reprod.* 2001;16(10):2066-2072.

[94] Karadag AS, Ertugrul DT, Tutal E, Akin KO. Short-term isotretinoin treatment decreases insulin-like growth factor-1 and insulin-like growth factor binding protein-3 levels: does isotretinoin affect growth hormone physiology? *Br. J. Dermatol.* 2010; 162(4):798-802.

[95] DeFronzo RA, Barzilai N, Simonson DC. Mechanism of metformin action in obese and lean noninsulin-dependent diabetic subjects. *J. Clin. Endocrinol. Metab.* 1991;73(6): 1294-1301.

[96] Pawelczyk L, Spaczynski RZ, Banaszewska B, Duleba AJ. Metformin therapy increases insulin-like growth factor binding protein-1 in hyperinsulinemic women with polycystic ovary syndrome. *Eur. J. Obstet. Gynecol. Reprod. Biol.* 2004;113(2):209-213.

[97] Jensterle M, Janez A, Mlinar B, Marc J, Prezelj J, Pfeifer M. Impact of metformin and rosiglitazone treatment on glucose transporter 4 mRNA expression in women with polycystic ovary syndrome. *Eur. J. Endocrinol.* 2008;158(6):793-801.

[98] Geisthovel F, Frorath B, Brabant G. Acarbose reduces elevated testosterone serum concentrations in hyperinsulinaemic premenopausal women: a pilot study. *Hum. Reprod.* 1996;11(11):2377-2381.

[99] Dreno B, Foulc P, Reynaud A, Moyse D, Habert H, Richet H. Effect of zinc gluconate on propionibacterium acnes resistance to erythromycin in patients with inflammatory acne: in vitro and in vivo study. *Eur. J. Dermatol.* 2005;15(3):152-155.

[100] Banudevi S, Senthilkumar K, Sharmila G et al. Effect of zinc on regulation of insulin-like growth factor signaling in human androgen-independent prostate cancer cells. *Clin. Chim. Acta.* 2010;411(10):172-178.

[101] Isard O, Knol AC, Ariès MF, Nguyen JM, Khammari A, Castex-Rizzi N, Dréno B. Propionibacterium acnes activates the IGF-1/IGF-1R system in the epidermis and induces keratinocyte proliferation. *J. Invest. Dermatol.* 2011;131(1):59-66.

In: Acne
Editor: Mohamed L. Elsaie
ISBN: 978-1-62618-358-2
© 2013 Nova Science Publishers, Inc.

Chapter V

Melanocortin-1 and -5 Receptors as Targets for Acne Therapy

Wen-Hwa Li[*], Li Zhang and Miri Seiberg
The Johnson and Johnson Skin Research Center,
CPPW, a unit of Johnson and Johnson Consumer Companies, Inc.,
Skillman, NJ, US

Abstract

Excessive sebum production is a key to the pathology of acne vulgaris, and the inhibition of sebum secretion predicts acne therapy outcome. Effective treatments for acne, such as isotretinoin and androgen modulators, inhibit sebaceous gland differentiation and sebum production. However, these agents also induce undesired effects, which limit their use in the clinics. Melanocortins, a series of neuropeptides derived from a parent pro-opiomelanocortin (POMC) molecule, bind to the melanocortin receptors. The melanocortin receptors 1 and 5 (MC1R, MC5R) are expressed in the sebaceous glands. MC1R has been associated with acne lesions, and MC5R is a marker of differentiated sebocytes. The production of sebaceous lipids is impaired in MC5R deficient mice, suggesting that MC5R is a regulator of sebum production. Therefore, the sebaceous gland melanocortin receptors were investigated as possible targets for acne therapy. A dual MC1R and MC5R antagonist

---

[*] Corresponding author: Wen-Hwa Li, E-mail: whli@its.jnj.com.

was shown to inhibit sebocyte differentiation in primary human sebocyte cultures, and to reduce sebum production in human skins transplanted onto immuno-deficient mice. These studies suggest that dual MC1R and MC5R antagonists may serve as potential topical therapeutic agents for sebaceous disorders with excess sebum, such as acne.

Keywords: Acne, MC1R, MC5R, melanocortin receptor 5 antagonist, sebaceous gland differentiation, sebocyte, sebum, lipids

Introduction

Acne is a chronic, multifactorial disease of the pilosebaceous unit, which affects millions of people worldwide. Although it is perceived as a disease of adolescence, acne can develop at any time, including neonatal, infantile and adult life [1]. Acne is manifested by the formation of skin lesions like whiteheads, blackheads, papules, pustules and cysts, which appear mainly on the face, shoulders and upper back. Although not life-threatening, acne affects the quality of life of patients by inducing psychological distress, hyperpigmented lesions, and permanent facial scarring [2]. The pathogenesis of acne has been attributed to four major pathways: excessive sebum production, follicular hyperkeratinization, hyperproliferation of *Propionibacterium acnes* (*P. acnes*), and inflammation [2-4]. The proliferation of sebocytes in the sebaceous gland and the elevation of sebum secretion have been associated with an increase in androgen activity [5, 6]. The relative contribution of each of these major pathological processes determines the type of the acne lesion, and the different mature lesions, therefore, respond to different therapies. It is desired to target an early event in the disease progression that would enable not only the treatment of multiple lesions, but also the prevention of new lesion initiation.

Acne Therapies and Their Adverse Effects

Current acne treatments aim to target as many pathological factors of the disease as possible, with topical over-the-counter monotherapies used for mild cases, and both topical and oral combination therapies prescribed for the more severe disease situations [reviewed in 2, 7]. Over-the-counter therapies include topical benzoyl peroxide or salicylic acid, and their continuous use at low levels may provide preventive measures, if side effects like skin dryness and irritation are tolerated. Topical retinoids, having both comedolytic and anti-inflammatory effects, are used as first line therapy for moderate acne, while combination therapies, such as a topical retinoid and an antimicrobial agent enable faster and greater clearing results for moderate to severe acne [2]. Topical retinoids could also be used for maintenance and preventive therapy, if side effects such as skin irritation, burning, scaling and dryness are tolerated [2].

Oral treatments, prescribed for the more severe disease states, include antibiotics, isotretinoin, and contraceptives [2, 8]. Oral antibiotics are used for patients with severe acne, acne of the back, or acne which is not responsive to topical treatment [9-11].

The long term use of low doses of antibiotics is not desired, as it may lead to antibiotic-resistance and loss of effectiveness [12]. Oral retinoid therapy, specifically oral isotretinoin, is the most effective therapy for moderate to severe inflammatory acne, including server nodulocystic scarring acne or acne resistant to other therapies. Oral isotretinoin affects several pathways involved in acne pathogenesis, with the greatest effect on sebum reduction [13]. However, using oral isotretinoin induces undesired effects like dermatitis, dry skin, secondary infection and photosensitivity, and increases the risk of teratogenic effects [review in 2, 14]. For women of childbearing age, therefore, oral isotretinoin treatment is used as a last resort, with enhanced contraceptive precautions [2]. Oral contraceptives, with a combination of an estrogen and progesterone, are effective in treating women with moderate-to-severe acne [2]. The combination therapy of an estrogen and cyproterone acetate reduced sebum secretion up to 75% [15]. However, contraceptives are not always desired for acne therapy, in particular when different birth control practices are preferred. Taken together, a common theme of effective acne therapies is the inhibition of sebum secretion, while their side effects and tolerability differ.

Clinically, sebum reduction correlates with the improvement of acne outcomes, such as total lesion count, inflammatory lesion count and acne severity grade [16]. Analyzing clinical data, Janiczek-Dolphin et al. [16] showed a significant correlation between sebum inhibition and acne outcomes across multiple studies which used unrelated therapies. Their conclusions confirm the notion that agents with sebum suppressing activity are useful in acne therapy.

Melanocortin Receptors in Skin

Melanocortins are neuropeptides derived from a parent POMC molecule, which bind to melanocortin receptors. The melanocortin system is implicated in numerous phenotypic traits, affecting various physiological and behavioral functions, such as sexual activity, aggressiveness, stress response, energy homeostasis, anti-inflammatory activities, and resistance to oxidative stress [review in 17, 18]. Of the five melanocortin receptors identified to date, four receptors, MC1R, MC2R, MC4R and MC5R, are expressed in human skin. MC1R is expressed in keratinocytes, dermal fibroblasts, melanocytes, sebaceous cells, hair follicle epithelial cells, sweat gland secretory and ductal epithelial cells, mast cells, adipocytes, and some periadnexal mesenchymal cells [19, 20]. MC1R has an important role in the regulation of skin and hair pigmentation [18, 21], immune and inflammation activities [22], and in interactions with the extracellular matrix to maintain skin homeostasis [23]. MC1R is expressed in both undifferentiated and differentiated sebocytes in the human sebaceous glands [24] and is expressed in sebaceous glands of acne skin at higher levels than those of normal skin [25]. MC2R expression is documented in human skin keratinocytes [26, 27]. MC2R has been implicated in human skin stress response [28] and in adipocytes' regulation of lipolysis [29, 30]. The immunoreactivity of MC4R is detected in human keratinocytes, melanocytes and dermal papillae cells [31, 32]. The role of MC4R in skin is not yet understood, and it is hypothesized to affect the regulation of pigmentation [31]. MC5R is found in the sebaceous glands, hair follicles, sweat glands and the epidermis [33]. MC5R is only detected in differentiated sebaceous cells but not in the basal, undifferentiated cells of the sebaceous glands. Therefore, it is considered a sebocyte differentiation marker [24]. MC5R might be involved in the regulation of sebaceous lipid production, since mice experimentally devoid of MC5R expression exhibited a defect in water repulsion, which resulted from a decrease in sebaceous lipid production [34, 35].

MC1R and Acne

The melanocortin alpha-melanocyte stimulating hormone (α-MSH) has been documented as a sebotrophic agent, a pigmentary hormone, and an inflammatory modulator [19, 36, 37]. α-MSH binds to all MCRs, with a high affinity to MC1R [19]. α-MSH is constitutively expressed at low levels in normal keratinocytes and is upregulated by ultraviolet (UV) light or by proinflammatory cytokines such as interleukin-1 (IL-1) [38], which are upregulated in acne [39-41]. Additionally, the expression of MC1R is upregulated by α-MSH [42] and by proinflammatory cytokines [43-45]. MC1R immunoreactivity is stronger in basal and peripheral differentiating sebocytes of lesional and non-lesional skins from acne patients, as compared to those of healthy skins [25]. In addition, keratinocytes in the non-involved and involved skin of the ductus seboglandularis had higher expression of MC1R than those of normal skin [25]. α-MSH induces the proliferation of HaCaT keratinocytes [46] but not of SZ95 sebocytes [47]. The combination of the α-MSH-induced keratinocyte proliferation with the increased immunoreactivity of MC1R might contribute to the extensive follicular hyperkeratinization in acne, suggesting that MC1R may act as a mediator of keratinocyte proliferation and differentiation.

MC5R and Sebaceous Lipid Regulation

In rodents, MC5R is the only MCR subtype that is expressed in secretary epithelia of exocrine glands, such as the Harderian, lacrimal, and preputial glands [34, 48-51]. Based on both in vitro and in vivo studies, Thody and coworkers suggested that α-MSH, which is a melanocortin, is a sebotrophic factor [52, 53]. They showed that when the neurointermediate lobes of the pituitary glands of rats were removed, the production of sebaceous lipids was reduced. The application of α-MSH and testosterone to hypophysectomized and castrated rats restored sebum secretion in these animals, suggesting a role for melanocortins in sebum production. Since α-MSH binds to all MCRs, no specific MCR was linked to sebum production in these studies. The first indication that MC5R might be involved in sebaceous lipid synthesis came from studies of MC5R deficient mice. These mice exhibited a decrease in sebaceous lipids production, which led to a defect in water repulsion and thermoregulation [34]. Additionally, POMC (the melanocortins precursor molecule)-deficient mice exhibited a similar defect in water repulsion and thermoregulation [54]. These studies support the hypothesis that, at least in rodents, the POMC peptides, which are the physiological ligands for MC5R, are involved in sebum regulation through MC5R.

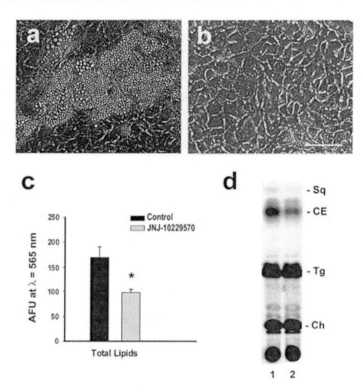

Figure 1. JNJ-10229570 inhibits sebaceous lipid production in vitro. (a) Differentiated human sebocytes induced by cholera toxin (CT) produce visible lipid droplets in culture. (b) Complete inhibition of sebocyte differentiation and lipid droplet production by JNJ-10229570 at 1 μM. (c) Quantification of neutral lipid production by Nile Red staining shows a significant reduction in total lipids production by sebocytes treated with JNJ-10229570. (d) HPTLC lipid profile of CT-induced (lane 1) and CT-induced and JNJ-10229570-treated sebocytes (lane 2) documents marked reduction in the sebaceous lipids squalene and cholesterol esters following JNJ-10229570 treatment. Ch=cholesterol, Tg=triglycerides, WE=wax esters, Sq=squalene. Bar=50 μm.

A Dual MC1R and MC5R Antagonist Can Inhibit Sebum Production

As described earlier, MC1R and MC5R are expressed in human sebaceous glands [19, 20, 24, 25, 33]; MC1R is expressed in sebaceous glands of acne skins at higher levels than those of normal skins [25]; sebaceous lipid production can be regulated by exogenous α-MSH [52, 53, 55]; and both

MC5R-deficient and POMC-deficient mice have reduced sebaceous lipid production [34, 54]. Taken together, these findings led to a search for agents with both MC1R and MC5R inhibitory activities. 5-phenylamino-2, 3-bis-(2-methoxyphenyl)-1, 2, 4-thiadiazoline (free base) (JNJ-10229570) [56, 57], was identified as an MC1R and MC5R antagonist that can reduce sebaceous lipid production [58].

JNJ-10229570 inhibited the binding of [^{125}I] NDP-α-MSH to membranes of cells overexpressing MC1R and MC5R, with IC$_{50}$s of about 200-300 nM [58]. JNJ-10229570 also inhibits cyclic adenosine monophosphate (cAMP) production from α-MSH-treated primary sebocytes [58], suggesting a functional antagonism in vitro.

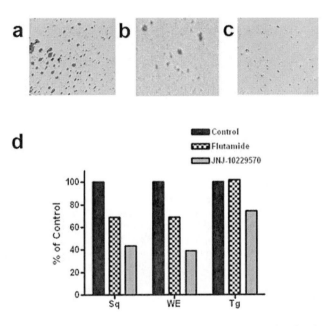

Figure 2. Topical treatment with JNJ-10229570 inhibits sebum secretion in vivo. (a-c) Human skins grafted onto SCID mice were topically treated with vehicle (a), flutamide (5%) (b), or JNJ-10229570 (0.05%) (c) for ~30 days. Sebum secretion is reduced in flutamide (b) and in JNJ-10229570 (c) treated skins, compared to vehicle control (a), as documented in images of skin surface lipids collected on SEBUTAPE®. (d) An HPTLC profile of the lipids synthesized de-novo in biopsies from the human/SCID study, cultured in the presence of ^{14}C-acetate. Phosphoimaging quantifying analysis of the HPTLC plates is presented as percent reduction relative to the total counts loaded. Both flutamide and JNJ-10229570 inhibited the synthesis of the sebaceous lipids squalene and wax esters as compared to the vehicle control, while triglyceride were minimally or not affected. Sq=squalene, WE=wax esters, Tg=triglycerides.

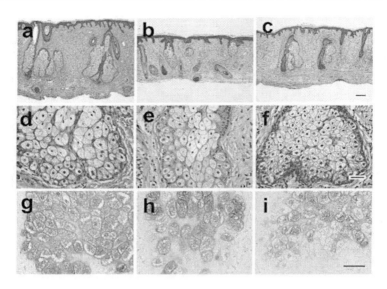

Figure 3. Topical treatment with JNJ-10229570 inhibits sebaceous glands differentiation. (a-i) Human skins grafted onto SCID mice were topically treated with vehicle (a, d, g), flutamide (5%) (b, e, h), or JNJ-10229570 (0.05%) (c, f, i) for ~30 days. Tissue sections were then stained histologically with HandE (a-f) or histochemically stained with epithelial-membrane antigen (EMA, g-i) to document the differentiation status of the sebaceous glands. Both flutamide (b, e) and JNJ-100229570 (c, f) treatments led to the development of smaller, and less lipid-loaded sebaceous glands as compared to the vehicle control (a, d). The sebaceous cells of the JNJ-100229570-treated skins (f) were somewhat smaller than those of the flutamide-treated skins (e), suggesting a stronger inhibition of sebocyte differentiation. EMA staining confirmed these results, documenting smaller and fewer EMA-stained sebocytes in JNJ-100229570-treated skins (i) as compared to the flutamide treatments (h) or vehicle-treated controls (g). These data suggest that JNJ-100229570 has the potential to inhibit sebocyte differentiation and sebum production in human, and therefore to provide a superior acne therapy. Bars=200 μm (a-c), 50 μm (d-i).

To evaluate the effect of JNJ-10229570 on sebocyte differentiation and lipid synthesis in vitro, human primary sebocyte cultures were induced to differentiation and then treated with JNJ-10229570 (see Figure 1). Lipid production in the treated sebocytes was documented by images of the lipid droplets within the cells, and was quantified by Nile Red staining of neutral lipids in the sebocyte culture, as described in [59, 60]. To investigate the de novo synthesis of the different lipid classes, the sebocyte cultures were incubated with [^{14}C]-acetate, and the different lipids (e.g. squalene, cholesterol esters, wax esters, triglycerides and cholesterol), were identified by high performance liquid chromatography (HPTLC), as described in [61]. These studies, shown in Figure 1, demonstrate that JNJ-10229570 inhibited sebaceous lipid production in vitro [58].

To study the effect of JNJ-10229570 on sebaceous lipid production in vivo, the model system used was of human skins transplanted onto server-combined-immunodeficient (SCID) mice [62]. Sebaceous glands were shown to develop in this model system, to resemble human sebaceous glands, and to secrete human sebum [63]. Flutamide, an acne therapeutic agent known to reduce sebum production in the clinic [64], was used to validate this model system. As shown in Figure 2, topical flutamide treatment led to a significant reduction in sebum secretion (documented by SEBUTAPE®), and to a marked reduction in the production of specific sebaceous lipids (documented by HPTLC), when compared to the controls. These results suggest that the human skin-SCID mouse system can detect changes in lipid production that are relevant to acne therapy.

Similar results were observed when the human skins grafted onto SCID mice were topically treated with JNJ-10229570 (see Figure 2). A marked decrease in sebum secretion was demonstrated by SEBUTAPE® as compared to the vehicle control, and reduced syntheses of squalene and wax esters were detected by HPTLC in JNJ-10229570-treated, [^{14}C]-acetate–labeled human skin biopsies [63]. When comparing to flutamide, these results suggest that JNJ-10229570 inhibits sebaceous lipid synthesis and sebum secretion to levels that are therapeutically effective in the clinics.

To follow on these finding, histological sections of human skin biopsies from the human skin-SCID mouse studies were evaluated for their sebaceous gland differentiation status. Both Flutamide and JNJ-10229570 inhibited sebaceous gland differentiation. As shown in Figure 3, the sebaceous glands and the sebaceous cells within the glands were smaller and less differentiated, and smaller lipid droplets were documented in the JNJ-10229570-treated human skin biopsies, as compared to the controls. Comparing the effects of flutamide and JNJ-10229570 in the same study, JNJ-10229570 was more effective than flutamide in reducing the size of the sebocytes, suggesting the possibility of a longer lasting therapeutic effect with JNJ-10229570. To further confirm the effect of these agents on the differentiation of the sebaceous glands, immuno-histochemical staining for the epithelial membrane antigen (EMA) was performed, as EMA is a marker of sebaceous cell differentiation [65]. As shown in Figure 3, there were fewer EMA-positive cells in sebaceous glands of JNJ-10229570-treated skin grafts than in those of vehicle-treated controls [58]. These results provide another indication that JNJ-10229570 reduces sebum production via its inhibitory effect on sebocyte differentiation.

The similar results obtained with flutamide confirmed the relevance of these studies to acne therapy.

Visual and histopathological analyses of the JNJ-10229570-treated skins did not show any adverse effects or skin architecture abnormalities [58]. In anticipation of pigmentary effects, both lightly- and darkly-pigmented human skins were evaluated in the human skin-SCID mouse studies. There was no visual change in skin colors, and image analysis of Fontana-Mason-stained sections revealed no trend of pigmentary changes. It remains to be studied why JNJ-10229570 exerts a significant effect on the MC5R pathway, with no significant effect on MC1R-induced pigmentation. These studies suggest the potential of MC5R antagonists and agents such as JNJ-10229570 in providing safe and effective acne therapy and prevention.

Conclusion

The effectiveness of acne treatments correlates with the inhibition of sebum production [16]. However, the most effective sebum secretion inhibitors available today induce numerous undesired effects [14]. Melanocortins are involved in the regulation of sebaceous lipids production [52, 53, 55]. MC5R was identified in lipid-laden, differentiated sebocytes, but not in the basal layer of human sebaceous glands [24], and MC5R-deficient mice showed a defect in sebaceous lipid production [34]. These findings suggest that MC5R antagonists might serve as acne therapies by inhibiting sebum production. JNJ-10229570, a dual MC1R and MC5R antagonist, was shown to inhibit sebocyte differentiation and to reduce sebum output in human skins transplanted onto immuno-compromised mice [58]. MC1R and MC5R antagonists such as JNJ-10229570 could, therefore, provide a safe and effective treatment of acne and other sebaceous gland disorders which are characterized by increased sebum production.

Acknowledgments

We would like to thank Dr. Magdalena Eisinger for leading the MC5R acne studies, and Michael Anthonavage, Dianne Rossetti, Drs. Apostolos Pappas, Qiuling Huang, Jimmy Xu and Nicole Molnar for their contribution to the discovery work. We are also grateful to Dr. Allen Reitz for chemistry support, to Dr. Druie Cavender for pharmacology advice and to Drs. Michael Southall, Claude Saliou and Curtis Cole for their critical reading of this manuscript.

References

[1] Friedlander, S. F., Baldwin, H. E., Mancini, A. J., Yan, A. C. and Eichenfield, L. F. (2011). The acne continuum: an age-based approach to therapy. *Semin. Cutan Med. Surg., 30(3 Suppl)*, S6-11.

[2] Williams, H. C., Dellavalle, R. P., and Garner, S. (2011). Acne vulgaris. *Lancet, 6736(11)*, 60321-60328.

[3] Kurokawa, I., Danby, F. W., Ju, Q., Wang, X., Xiang, L. F., Xia, L., Chen, W., Nagy, I., Picardo, M., Suh, D. H., Ganceviciene, R., Schagen, S., Tsatsou, F., and Zouboulis, C. C. (2009). New developments in our understanding of acne pathogenesis and treatment. *Exp. Dermatol., 18(10)*, 821-832.

[4] Makrantonaki, E., Ganceviciene, R., and Zouboulis, C. C. (2011). An update of the role of the sebaceous gland in the pathogenesis of acne. *Dermato-Endocrinology, 3(1)*, 41-49.

[5] Pochi, P. E., and Strauss, J. S. (1969). Sebaceous gland response in man to the administration of testosterone, delta-4-androstenedione, and dehydroisoandrosterone. *J. Invest. Dermatol., 52*, 32–36.

[6] Akamatsu, H., Zouboulis, C. C., and Orfanos, C. E. (1992). Control of human sebocyte proliferation in vitro by testosterone and 5-DHT is dependent on the localization of the sebaceous glands. *J. Invest. Dermatol., 99*, 509-511.

[7] Zaenglein, A. L., and Thiboutot, D. M. (2006). Expert committee recommendations for acne management. *Pediatrics, 118(3)*, 1188-1199.

[8] Strauss, J. S., Krowchuck, D. P., Leyden, J. J., Lucky, A. W., Shalita, A. R., Siegfried, E. C., Thiboutot, D. M., Van Voorhees, A. S., Beutner, K. A., Sieck, C. K., Bhushan, R., and American Academy of Dermatology/American Academy of Dermatology Association. (2007). Guidelines of care for acne vulgaris management. *J. Am. Acad. Dermatol., 56(4)*, 651–663.

[9] Ozolins, M., Eady, E. A., Avery, A. J., Cunliffe, W. J., Po, A. L., O'Neill, C., Simpson, N. B., Walters, C. E., Carnegie, E., Lewis, J. B., Dada, J., Haynes, M., Williams, K., and Williams, H. C. (2004).

Comparison of five antimicrobial regimens for treatment of mild to moderate infl ammatory facial acne vulgaris in the community: randomized controlled trial. *Lancet, 364*, 2188–2195.

[10] Ochsendorf, F. (2010). Minocycline in Acne Vulgaris: Benefits and Risks. *Am. J. Clin. Dermatol., 11 (5)*, 327-341.

[11] Maffeis, L., and Veraldi, S. (2010). Minocycline in the treatment of acne: latest findings. *G. Ital. Dermatol. Venereol., 145(3)*, 425-429.

[12] Eady, A. E., Cove, J. H., and Layton, A. M. (2003). Is antibiotic resistance in cutaneous propionibacteria clinically relevant? Implications of resistance for acne patients and prescribers. *Am. J. Clin. Dermatol., 4*, 813–831.

[13] Gollnick, H., Cunliffe, W., Berson, D., Dreno, B., Finlay, A., Leyden, J. J., Shalita, A. R., and Thiboutot, D. Global Alliance to Improve Outcomes in Acne. (2003). Management of acne, a report from a global alliance to improve outcomes in acne. *J. Am. Acad. Dermatol., 49*, S1–37.

[14] Kontaxakis, V. P., Skourides, D., Ferentinos, P., Havaki-Kontaxaki, B. J., and Papadimitriou, G. N. (2009). Isotretinoin and psychopathology: a review. *Ann. Gen. Psychiatry, 8*, 2.

[15] Hughes, B. R., and Cunliffe, W. J. (1994). A prospective study of the effect of isotretinoin in the follicular reservoir and sustainable sebum excretion rate in patients with acne. *Arch. Dermatol., 130*, 315–318.

[16] Janiczek-Dolphin, N., Cook, J., Thiboutot, D., Harness, J., and Clucas, A. (2010). Can sebum reduction predict acne outcome? *Br. J. Dermatol., 163(4)*, 683-688.

[17] Gantz, I., and Fong, T. M. (2003). The melanocortin system. *Am. J. Physiol. Endocrinol. Metab., 284(3)*, E468-474.

[18] Roulin, A., and Ducrest, A. L. (2011). Association between melanism, physiology and behavior: a role for the melanocortin system. *Eur. J. Pharmacol., 660(1)*, 226-233.

[19] Bohm, M., Schiller, M., Stander, S., Seltmann, H., Li, Z., Brzoska, T., Metze, D., Schioth, H. B., Skottner, A., Seiffert, K., Zouboulis, C.C., and Luger, T. A. (2002). Evidence for expression of melanocortin-1 receptor in human sebocytes in vitro and in situ. *J. Invest. Dermatol., 118*, 533–539.

[20] Bohm, M., Luger, T. A., Tobin, D. J., and Garcia-Borron, J. C. (2006). Melanocortin receptor ligands: new horizons for skin biology and clinical dermatology. *J. Invest. Dermatol., 126*, 1966–1975.

[21] Dessinioti, C., Antoniou, C., Katsambas, A., and Stratigos, A. J. (2011). Melanocortin 1 receptor variants: functional role and pigmentary associations. *Photochem. Photobiol., 87(5)*, 978-987.

[22] Brzoska, T., Luger, T. A., Maaser, C., Abels, C., and Bohm, M. (2008). Alpha-melanocytestimulating hormone and related tripeptides: biochemistry, antiinflammatory and protective effects in vitro and in vivo, and future perspectives for the treatment of immune-mediated inflammatory diseases. *Endocr. Rev., 29*, 581–602.

[23] Bohm, M., Raghunath, M., Sunderkotter, C., Schiller, M., Stander, S., Brzoska, T., Cauvet, T., Schioth, H. B., Schwarz, T., and Luger, T. A. (2004). Collagen metabolism is a novel target of the neuropeptide alpha-melanocyte-stimulating hormone. *J. Biol. Chem., 279*, 6959–6966.

[24] Zhang, L., Li, W. H., Anthonavage, M., and Eisinger, M. (2006). Melanocortin-5 receptor: a marker of human sebocyte differentiation. *Peptides, 27*, 413–420.

[25] Ganceviciene, R., Graziene, V., Bohm, M., and Zouboulis, C. C. (2007). Increased in situ expression of melanocortin-1 receptor in sebaceous glands of lesional skin of patients with acne vulgaris. *Exp. Dermatol., 16(7)*, 547-552.

[26] Slominski, A., Ermak, G., and Mihm, M. (1996). ACTH receptor, CYP11A1, CYP17 and CYP21A2 genes are expressed in skin. *J. Clin. Endocrinol. Metab., 81*, 2746–2749.

[27] Moustafa, M., Szabo, M., Ghanem, G. E., Morandini, R., Kemp, E. H., MacNeil, S., and Haycock, J. W. (2002). Inhibition of tumor necrosis factor-alpha stimulated NFkappaB/p65 in human keratinocytes by alpha-melanocyte stimulating hormone and adrenocorticotropic hormone peptides. *J. Invest. Dermatol., 119*, 1244–1253.

[28] Slominski, A., Wortsman, J., Luger, T., Paus, R., and Solomon, S. (2000). Corticotropin releasing hormone and proopiomelanocortin involvement in the cutaneous response to stress. *Physiol. Rev., 80*, 979–1020.

[29] Boston, B. A., and Cone, R. D. (1996). Characterization of melanocortin receptor subtype expression in murine adipose tissues and in the 3T3-L1 cell line. *Endocrinology, 137*, 2043–2050.

[30] Xue, B., Moustaid, N., Wilkison, W. O., and Zemel, M. B. (1998). The agouti gene product inhibits lipolysis in human adipocytes via a Ca^{2+}-dependent mechanism. *FASEB J., 12*, 1391–1396.

[31] Spencer, J. D., and Schallreuter, K. U. (2009). Regulation of pigmentation in human epidermal melanocytes by functional high-

affinity beta-melanocyte stimulating hormone/melanocortin-4 receptor signaling. *Endocrinology, 150*, 1250–1258.

[32] Bohm, M., and Luger, T. A. (2004). Melanocortins in fibroblast biology–current update and future perspective for dermatology. *Exp. Dermatol., 13 (Suppl 4)*, 16–21.

[33] Thiboutot, D., Sivarajah, A., Gilliland, K., Cong, Z., and Clawson, G. (2000). The melanocortin 5 receptor is expressed in human sebaceous glands and rat preputial cells. *J. Invest. Dermatol., 115*, 614–619.

[34] Chen, W., Kelly, M. A., Opitz-Araya, X., Thomas, R. E., Low, M. J., and Cone, R. D. (1997). Exocrine gland dysfunction in MC5-R-deficient mice: evidence for coordinated regulation of exocrine gland function by melanocortin peptides. *Cell, 91*, 789–798.

[35] Cone, R. D. (2006). Studies on the physiological functions of the melanocortin system. *Endocr. Rev., 27*, 736–749.

[36] Lipton, J. M., and Catania, A. (1997). Antiinflammatory actions of the neuroimmunomodulator α-MSH. *Immunol. Today, 18*, 140-145.

[37] Bhardwaj, R. S., Schwarz, A., Becher, E., Mahnke, K., Aragane, Y., Schwarz, T., and Luger, T. A. (1996). Proopiomelanocortin-derived peptides induce IL-10 production in human monocytes. *J. Immunol., 156*, 2517-2521.

[38] Schauer, E., Trautinger, F., Kock, A., Schwarz, A., Bhardwaj, R., Simon, M., Ansel, J. C., Schwarz, T., and Luger, T. A. (1994). Proopiomelanocortin-derived peptides are synthesized and released by human keratinocytes. *J. Clin. Invest., 93*, 2258-2262.

[39] Ingham, E., Eady, E. A., Goodwin, C. E., Cove, J. H., and Cunliffe, W. J. (1992). Proinflammatory levels of interleukin-1 alpha-like bioactivity are present in the majority of open comedones in acne vulgaris. *J. Invest. Dermatol., 98*, 895–901.

[40] Jeremy, A., Holland, D., Roberts, S., Thomson, K., and Cunliffe, W. (2003). Inflammatory events are involved in acne lesion initiation. *J. Invest. Dermatol., 121*, 20–27.

[41] Boehm, K. D., Yun, J. K., Strohl, K. P., and Elmets, C. A. (1995). Messenger RNAs for the multifunctional cytokines interleukin-1 alpha, interleukin-1 beta and tumor necrosis factor-alpha are present in adnexal tissues and in dermis of normal human skin. *Exp. Dermatol., 4(6)*, 335-341.

[42] Rouzaud, F., Annereau, J. P., Valencia, J. C., Costin, G. E., and Hearing, V. J. (2003). Regulation of melanocortin 1 receptor expression at the

mRNA and protein levels by its natural agonist and antagonist. *FASEB J., 17*, 2154-2156.
[43] Bhardwaj, R., Becher, E., Mahnke, K., Hartmeyer, M., Schwarz, T., Scholzen, T., and Luger, T. A. (1997). Evidence for the differential expression of the functional alpha-melanocyte stimulating hormone receptor MC-1 on human monocytes. *J. Immunol., 158*, 3378–3384.
[44] Hartmeyer, M., Sholzen, T., Becher, E., Bhardwaj, R., Schwarz, T., and Luger T. A. (1997). Human dermal microvascular endothelial cells express the melanocortin receptor type 1 and produce increased levels of IL-8 upon stimulation with alpha-melanocyte stimulating hormone. *J. Immunol., 159*, 1930–1937.
[45] Ganceviciene, R., Bohm, M., Fimmel, S., and Zouboulis, C. C. (2009). The role of neuropeptides in the multifactorial pathogenesis of acne vulgaris. *Dermatoendocrinology, 1*, 170–176.
[46] Orel, L., Simon, M., Karlseder , J., Bhardwaj, R., Trautinger, F., Schwarz, T., and Luger, T. A. (1997). Alpha-melanocyte stimulating hormone downregulates differentiation driven heat shock protein 70 expression in keratinocytes. *J. Invest. Dermatol., 108*, 401–405.
[47] Zouboulis, C. C., Xia, L., Akamatsu, H., Seltmann, H., Fritsch, M., Hornemann, S., Rühl, R., Chen, W., Nau, H., and Orfanos, C. E. (1998). The human sebocyte culture model provides new insights into development and management of seborrhoea and acne. *Dermatology, 196*, 21–31.
[48] Griffon, N., Mignon, V., Facchinetti, P., Diaz, J., Schwartz, J., and Sokoloff, P. (1994). Molecular cloning and characterization of the rat fifth melanocortin receptor. *Biochem. Biophys. Res. Commun., 200*, 1007–1014.
[49] Labbe, O., Desarnaud, F., Eggerickx, D., Vassart, G., and Parmentier, M. (1994). Molecular cloning of a mouse melanocortin 5 receptor gene widely expressed in peripheral tissues. *Biochemistry, 33*, 4543–4549.
[50] Gantz, I., Shimoto, Y., Konda, Y., Miwa, H., Dickinson, C. J., and Yamada, T. (1994). Molecular cloning, expression, and characterization of a fifth melanocortin receptor. *Biochem. Biophys. Res. Commun., 200*, 1214–1220.
[51] van der Kraan, M., Adan, R. A., Entwistle, M. L., Gispen, W. H., Burbach, J. P., and Tatro, J. B. (1998). Expression of melanocortin-5 receptor in secretary epithelia supports a functional role in exocrine and endocrine glands. *Endocrinology, 139*, 2348–2355.

[52] Thody, A. J., and Shuster, S. (1975). Control of sebaceous gland function in the rat by alphamelanocyte-stimulating hormone. *J. Endocrinol., 64*, 503–510.
[53] Thody, A. J., Cooper, M. F., Bowden, P. E., Meddis, D., and Shuster, S. (1976). Effect of alpha-melanocyte stimulating hormone and testosterone on cutaneous and modified sebaceous glands in the rat. *J. Endocrinol., 71*, 279–288.
[54] Yaswen, L., Diehl, N., Brennan, M. B., and Hochgeschwender, U. (1999). Obesity in the mouse model of pro-opiomelanocortin deficiency responds to peripheral melanocortin. *Nat. Med., 5*, 1066–1070.
[55] Zhang, L., Anthonavage, M., Huang, Q., Li, W. H., and Eisinger, M., (2003). Proopiomelanocortin peptides and sebogenesis. *Ann. N. Y. Acad. Sci., 994*, 154–161.
[56] Pan, K., and Reitz, A. B. (2002). The synthesis of aminobenzothiazoles from 2, 3-biaryl-5 anilino-Δ3–1, 2, 4-thiadiazolines. *Synth. Commun., 33*, 2053–2060.
[57] Pan, K., Scott, M. K., Lee, D. H., Fitzpatrick, L. J., Crooke, J. J., Rivero, R. A., Rosenthal, D. I. Vaidya, A. H., Zhao, B., and Reitz, A. B. (2003). 2, 3-Diaryl-5-anilino[1, 2, 4]thiadiazoles as melanocortin MC4 receptor agonists and their effects on feeding behavior in rats. *Bioorg. Med. Chem., 11*, 185–192.
[58] Eisinger, M., Li, W. H., Anthonavage, M., Pappas, A., Zhang, L., Rossetti, D., Huang, Q., and Seiberg, M. (2011). A melanocortin receptor 1 and 5 antagonist inhibits sebaceous gland differentiation and the production of sebum-specific lipids. *J. Dermatol. Sci., 63(1)*, 23-32.
[59] McMillian, M. K., Grant, E. R., Zhong, Z., Parker, J. B., Li, L., Zivin, R. A., Burczynski, M. E., and Johnson, M. D. (2001). Nile red binding to HepG2 cells: an improved assay for in vitro studies of hepatosteatosis. *In Vitr. Mol. Toxicol., 14*, 177-190.
[60] Zouboulis, C. C., Seltmann, H., Hiroi, N., Chen, W., Young, M., Oeff, M., Scherbaum, W. A., Orfanos, C. E., McCann, S. M., and Bornstein, S. R. (2002). Corticotropin-releasing hormone: An autocrine hormone that promotes lipogenesis in human sebocytes. *PNAS, 99*, 7148-7153.
[61] Pappas, A., Anthonavage, M., and Gordon, J. S. (2002). Metabolic fate and selective utilization of major fatty acids in human sebaceous gland. *J. Invest. Dermatol., 118*, 164–171.
[62] Juhasz, I., Murphy, G. F., Yan, H. C., Herlyn, M., and Albelda, S. M. (1993). Regulation of extracellular matrix proteins and integrin cell

substratum adhesion receptors on epithelium during cutaneous human wound healing in vivo. *Am. J. Pathol., 143*, 1458–1469.

[63] Eisinger, M., Li, W. H., Rossetti, D., Anthonavage, M., and Seiberg, M. (2010). Sebaceous gland regeneration in human skin xenografts. *J. Invest. Dermatol., 130*, 2131–2133.

[64] Wang, H-S, Wang, T-H, and Soong, Y-K. (1999). Low dose flutamide in the treatment of Acne Vulgaris in women with or without oligomenorrhea or amenorrhea. *Chang Gung Med. J., 22*, 423-432.

[65] Latham, J. A., Redfern, C. P., Thody, A. J., and De Kretser, T. A. (1989). Immunohistochemical markers of human gland differentiation. *J. Histochem. Cytochem., 37*, 729–734.

In: Acne
Editor: Mohamed L. Elsaie

ISBN: 978-1-62618-358-2
© 2013 Nova Science Publishers, Inc.

Chapter VI

Psychosocial and Emotional Aspects of Acne: The Need for a Psychosomatic Approach to Management

K. Stephen and A. G. Affleck[*]
Ninewells Hospital, Dundee, Scotland, United Kingdom

"There is no single disease which causes more psychic trauma, more maladjustment pushing parents and children apart, more general insecurity and feelings of inferiority and greater sums of psychic suffering than does acne vulgaris" [1]

Abstract

Acne usually presents in adolescents, a time of physical change and emotional instability. This extra change in self-image can compromise self-esteem and self-consciousness further. In individuals with extra risk factors and reduced resilience factors, the coping mechanism can be tipped out of balance leading to psychological and functional morbidity.

---

[*] E-mail: andrew.affleck@nhs.net. Tel: +44(0)1382 660111 Ext: 33004, Fax: +44(0)1382 633916.

It has long been recognised that in some people with acne, stress appears to contribute towards flare ups. Such stress-responders may benefit from relaxation training and other aspects of stress management. There is a spectrum of emotional sequelae secondary to acne: some individuals appear to be extremely stoical and resistant to emotional morbidity with positive coping mechanisms, even with objectively severe acne on physical examination; other individuals appear to be more prone to emotional morbidity even when objectively there is mild acne; the reasons for this are complex and have been addressed in several studies. Unfavourable coping is found in 5 associated psychiatric disorders, namely: adjustment disorder, depression, social phobia and anxiety disorder. Eating disorder and Body Dysmorphic Disorder. Therefore, it is best practice to assess patients who have acne for such associated psychological comorbidities to achieve maximum benefit and minimise risk to the patient. When psychiatric comorbidity is present, it should be addressed and treated and when necessary, referral to a specialist in mental health is desirable. A psychosomatic approach to a new patient with acne based on the biopsychosocial model of illness is desirable. Further assessment and treatment is individualised to that patient. Simple measures like use of SUbjective Discomfort Scores (SUDS), self reported by the patient, assessing general well being, anxiety, depression and stress are a good starting point. Core communication skills and basic counselling to generate a strong rapport with the patient, demonstrating empathy and exploring the impact on quality of life and the patients perceived ideas and illness perception is useful. Most patients with acne do not have severe associated psychological morbidity and one needs to avoid "psychologicalising" them, but a minority do and these are the at-risk patients that we need to identify, as unfortunately suicide is a recognised association in such patients. The use of validated general health questionnaires, mental health questionnaires and dermatology-specific questionnaires can also help in information gathering. Acne excoriee can be helped with a combined therapeutic approach including behavioural therapy habit reversal training. Time is a limiting factor in busy clinics, however efforts should be made to allow for more time for individual patients who have unmet needs, and a multidisciplinary approach using perhaps an experienced nurse to listen to, and talk with appropriate patients in a counselling capacity or indeed referral to colleagues in Clinical Psychology or liaison Psychiatry when necessary. A motivated, trained and knowledgeable Dermatologist can help patients who have acne and significant psychosocial detriment with a well thought out, planned, holistic approach using conventional topical therapy, oral therapy, including isotretinoin, and psychological therapy whether it be supportive, motivational or cognitive-behavioural and occasionally psychopharmacological therapy. This psychosomatic approach will result in better patient outcome with increased patient satisfaction.

Introduction

Acne usually presents in adolescents, a time of physical change and emotional instability. [2] This extra change in self-image can compromise self-esteem and self-consciousness further. In individuals with extra risk factors and reduced resilience factors, the coping mechanism can be tipped out of balance leading to psychological, emotional and functional morbidity. [2] It is generally accepted that adolescents, who represent the largest proportion of acne sufferers, are the most vulnerable to the negative effects of the disease. [3] Theoretically, adolescents who have had difficult childhood experiences and as a result are unable to establish a good body image and a positive self esteem, are at particular risk of psychological deterioration with the onset of acne. [4] The consequences of a decreased self esteem with associated distortion of self image include depressive symptoms, social withdrawal, difficulty with family and peer relationships, deterioration in academic performance, unemployment, anger, frustration and embarrassment. [2] In severely affected individuals depressive symptoms may contribute towards disciplinary issues and severe family conflict.

A holistic approach to the assessment and management of the patient with acne will help identify those in need of extra support and individually tailored talking, listening and guiding therapy.

The physical pathogenesis of acne is discussed elsewhere. Physical treatments aim to reverse the multiple physical aetiologies at play. Early physical treatment may reduce psychoemotional morbidity; the common consensus is that treatment should be started without delay in any patient to minimise progression to inflammatory acne and potential scarring which can have significant impact on the patient's social functioning and even employment opportunities [2, 3] However, before treatment is initiated the patient's expectations regarding the treatment must be dealt with, as they often have too high an expectation of therapy leading to poor adherence. If not seeing the desired results in the time frame they expect, the patient often stops treatment assuming that it is not working. Patients may discontinue treatment because quick results are not seen and so they presume the treatment is ineffective. There are many effective medical treatments for acne available and if used correctly, an improvement in psychological health and quality of life is often seen. [5] Accordingly, the need for good doctor-patient communication and treatment education is essential to ensure patients achieve optimum concordance with suggested treatment regimens and that patients with poor coping strategies or co-morbid psychopathology do not lose hope with, and discontinue, their treatment, which in turn may lead to further negative psychological outcomes. Motivational techniques and an increased frequency of consultations can help optimise adherence to treatment. [6]

Acne has a genetic basis but this can be influenced by external factors including emotions and stress. Therefore it can be described as being multifactorial, and so a holistic approach, assessing both physical and emotional features is desirable. [2] Acne affects the person in a unique way and this varies enormously from person to person. The affect on the person is dependent on the pre-existing psychological makeup. The psychology of adolescence is very complicated and has been studied extensively over the years – this period can exhibit feelings of inferiority, emotional immaturity and instability. The onset of acne can worsen these negative emotions. Each person with acne has a unique experience and this is influenced by many complex factors, including personality, perceptions, previous experiences and social support or lack of. Most adolescents in the Western world have acne for some time which is mostly mild and self-limiting, requiring no medical treatment or self-treated with over-the-counter preparations. Most people have only mild and transient emotional upset with no long lasting morbidity. However, in a minority, the emotional impact can be devastating and long term. (Table 1).

Table 1. Potential Negative Emotional Impact of Acne (feelings)

anxiety
sadness
frustration
anger
annoyance
contempt
disgust
fear
doubt
envy
ashamed
despair
disappointment
reduced confidence
self-consciousness
embarrassment
hurt
guilt

Secondary scarring can be a permanent reminder of previous emotional distress. Therefore acne should never be trivialised as it appears to still be by some people including family doctors with attempts at reassuring comments such as "It is only acne – it will soon go away" and an apparent reluctance to refer to secondary care (personal observation).

Psychological disturbance is now considered to be a secondary event whereas in the past there was a school of thought that considered acne to be exacerbated or caused by psychopathology. This is now generally disregarded, although there may be a small subset of patients with chronic treatment resistant acne who may see physical improvement with the addition of non-medical treatment e.g. insight-orientated psychotherapy as reported by Koblenzer [7] and hypnosis and relaxation therapy as reported by Shenefelt. [8]

Historical Aspects

Historically, acne was considered to be associated with sexual factors and specifically that satisfaction of sexual needs could be curative. Attempts were made to categorise certain acne personality types but as acne is so common, affecting approximately 80% of adolescents, it became clear that no particular personality type is predisposed. [9] Some authors, influenced by the work of Freud, considered acne as an example of a dermatological conversion symptom formed due to unresolved inner conflict. Kenyon stated in his paper in 1966 that the literature at the time was "awash with vague generalisations, anecdotes and speculations and almost totally lacking in any controlled investigations". [10]

In the 1950s Obermayer, a pioneer in the emotional aspects of skin disease stressed the potential impact of acne on the individual "in which the necessity for supportive psychotherapy cannot be overemphasized". [9] He comments further that, "A great deal of harm is done by the physician who neglects to act accordingly to this concept". [9] However, Obermayers's words of wisdom did not appear to be heard by all as shown in a review paper from 1969, which had no mention of potential psychoemotional or behavioural impact of patients with acne.

Shuster showed in 1978 that acne caused a significant decline in self image, especially objectively severe acne and more noticeable in women. [12]

This negative effect appeared to be greater than 2 other common inflammatory skin diseases – eczema and psoriasis.

The acne disability index developed in 1989 by Motley and Finlay is a simple short 5-item questionnaire which patients can complete which can give a pointer towards the degree of emotional and practical problems related to acne.[13, 14] The same study cleverly looked at how much people were prepared to pay for a hypothetical cure. Interestingly, this amount did not correlate with the objective acne severity but did correlate with the Acne Disability Index. This highlights the individual experience of a person with acne and emphasises that without an extended history into psychosocial and emotional factors and effect on quality of life, one cannot judge the overall impact of acne on that person.

Acne as an Example of a Biopsychosocial Model of Illness

Fava, in an excellent review, defines psychosomatic medicine as, "a comprehensive interdisciplinary framework for:

1. Assessment of psychosocial factors affecting individual vulnerability, course, and outcome of any type of disease
2. Holistic consideration of patient care in clinical practice
3. Integration of psychological therapies in the prevention, treatment, and rehabilitation of medical disease" [15]

It would appear obvious to use this approach in skin disease with significant impact on the person's life eg. acne.

The referral to talking therapies and the role for psychosomatic approach in patient management has been suggested numerous times in the reviewed literature; however this still does not seem to be a standard practice in dermatology [2, 3, 4].

It has been reported that, amongst patients referred to a liaison psychiatrist within a dermatology clinic, psychiatric intervention resulted in clinical improvement in most of those followed up. [16] It is also suggested that dermatologists should familiarise themselves with at least the basics of superficial psychotherapy and psycho pharmaceutical therapy, which may be needed in addition to topical and systemic acne treatments in order to treat the patient holistically for the optimum result, not just the skin condition. [17]

The psychosomatic approach helps to generate rapport and engagement. The use of core communication skills allows a therapeutic trusting relationship to develop. Basic counselling techniques demonstrating empathy is needed.

Table 2. Potential negative Psychological Factors in Acne (thoughts / beliefs)

unattractiveness
unacceptability to self and others
self-disgust
self-hatred
perceived inferiority to others
perceived ugliness
unlovable
unworthy
repulsive to others
flawed
imperfect
unclean
unable to cope
suicidal ideation

Patients with acne should be encouraged to express their feelings verbally or in the form of written disclosure / emotional diary. This "normalising" of perceived emotions can be therapeutic in itself and help in the adjustment process. Patients should be informed that many people with acne describe a similar range of emotions. Patients may disclose their negative beliefs about acne (Table 2) and again it can be helpful to discuss these thoughts in an open, non-judgmental way.

Use of hypnotherapy with positive imagery, biofeedback and Insight orientated psychotherapy is practised by only a few psychodermatologists with further qualifications and training. These advanced techniques are not widely available but may help some patients with chronic treatment-resistant acne. [4, 7, 8]

The art of psychocutaneous medicine is covered in detail in other recognized texts which the enthusiastic reader can refer to. [18,19, 20]

Stigma

Stigma is a complicated topic which occurs as a result of negative labelling ie. a negative social response of an individual or group to a physical, psychological or social difference in another person. Several definitions exist – "a distinguishing personal trait that is perceived as or actually is physically, socially, or psychologically disadvantageous" [21] or "a sign, mark, feature, indicator of something, which generally has a negative connotation". [22] Being visibly different is a common cause of stigma and so having a skin disease eg. acne, may be problematic and result in "public humiliation and social disgrace". The patient with acne may deviate psychologically and socially from others and so lead to further negative labelling. Stigma can be discreditable (not widely known eg. hidden truncal acne) or discrediting (cannot be hidden due to obvious visibility eg. facial acne). Discreditable stigma may have an important effect on the person's own behaviour eg. avoiding swimming but as it is concealed it does not affect the behaviour of others. In contrast, with discrediting stigma, people may respond to the visible difference rather than the person. Negative judgements and actions can be made with resultant profound psychoemotional and social effects. Ritvo et al. performed a study comparing how adults and teenagers evaluated teenagers with acne compared to those with smooth clear skin. [23] Participants were invited by email to complete on-line surveys. 1002 adults aged18 or over and 1006 teenagers were enrolled. Each respondent was asked about 3 randomly selected pictures which were a combination of either 1 clear and 2 acne or 2 clear and 1 acne. Acne was not specifically mentioned during the perception survey. Respondents were also asked about their own experiences with acne in a second survey. Most teenagers and adults (65%, 75%) noticed the skin first for photos of a person with acne compared with only 14% Teenagers and 16% adults for photos of a person with clear skin.

Teenagers with clear skin were thought to be:

"Happy, healthy, intelligent, self-confident, fun, trustworthy, creative, popular, cool, athletic, and outspoken"

Teenagers with acne were thought to be:

"Shy, introverted, lonely, nerdy, stressed, unhealthy, unkempt, boring and rebellious".

The majority of both teens and adults thought the way they look is important. 55% of teens and 45% of adults felt that getting acne was the most difficult aspect of puberty. 64% of teens were embarrassed by it however only 17% of parents found their teenager's acne a source of embarrassment.

Teenagers with acne reported lower self-confidence or shyness, difficulty finding dates, problems making friends, challenges with school and trouble getting a job.

Roosta and colleagues, sampled 336 young adults attending a University with a web-based survey. [24] Multivariant modelling was used to determine if acne resulted in perceived stigma. They found that the likelihood of experiencing perceived stigma was 3.19 times higher for those with acne, compared to those without acne (95% CI 2.41- 4.22, P < 0.001). Respondents who had eczema were less likely to experience perceived stigma − 1.6 times higher than controls without eczema. They conclude that acne may have a stronger relationship with perceived stigma than eczema, perhaps because of its greater visibility on the body.

These studies support the existing evidence on the stigmatising effect of acne. It appears that unfounded judgements are commonly made. As Lowe states, "education of the general public and of future doctors is essential in order to remove the stigma of this common condition". [25]

School and University-based activities should be recommended to support those with skin disease.

Psychosocial Impact of Acne − the Role of Confounding Psychological Factors

Psychosocial functioning is determined by many different interacting factors, including self-esteem, psychopathology, body image related problems and perceived stress. [26] The majority of previous studies on the psychoemotional impact of acne and its effect on quality of life on are semi-quantitative analyses of patients' responses to surveys and questionnaires. [27, 28, 29]

Medansky et.al found in a study of 145 patients, that anxiety levels in people with acne were the same as controls from the normal population. [30] Indeed most patients also had normal self esteem and perceived peer popularity. There have been some other more recent studies, again which have shown no significant emotional detriment, but there are contrasting results from other studies showing significant anxiety and reduced self esteem, embarrassment, self consciousness and social isolation. Therefore, with the apparent contradictory results from studies it is clear that generalisation is not helpful.

Krejci – Manwaring and colleagues, performed a survey-based study to investigate whether personality trait dispositional social sensitivity could be associated with the adverse social impact of acne. [31] 479 people with acne responded and were classified as either high or low social sensitivity. The degrees of acne severity was significantly associated with poorer social outcomes and quality of life, and in women, higher social sensitivity was independently associated with poorer outcome (P < 0.05) while for men, higher social sensitivity interacted with acne severity and was associated with worse social outcomes and quality of life (P < 0.05). They conclude that dispositional social sensitivity is an independent psychological factor associated with poorer social functioning and quality of life in acne patients.

Appearance Perception and Body Image

Body image is "a multidimensional construct that comprises perceptions and attitude towards one's own body, mainly but not entirely limited to the physical appearance". [32] The 2 main parts of this construct are evaluation (body satisfaction) and investment in one's appearance. Self-esteem can be described as "the attitude of worth in which the person holds himself or herself and the value one accords to oneself". Self-image refers to concepts of self-esteem and body image, important dimensions throughout life especially during adolescence. Research has shown an increase prevalence of negative body image, especially amongst women, which may be in part driven by cosmetic and advertising industries with a constant use of images (often facial) showing a perfect appearance. [32] In modern society these ideas are constantly reinforced to the extent that they may become accepted values. It is therefore perhaps unsurprising that in susceptible individuals, who perhaps have acne, secondary emotional morbidity occurs, including low mood and reduced self-esteem. Women are probably more vulnerable to this due the gender biased cultural socialisation.

Beauty ideals and body concerns have been shown to vary amongst different cultures. Individuals may also be more vulnerable at specific transitional periods in life e.g. puberty (as in acne), early childhood, pregnancy and mid or later life.

Cash has done much work in body image and developed the Body Image Quality of Life Inventory (BLQLI) in 2002. [32] This is a self-reported short questionnaire with 19 items reflecting specific domains, including day to day emotions, self-esteem, sexuality, social relationships, routine exercise, grooming habits and life satisfaction. Many of these domains are covered in other validated self-report questionnaires, including DLQI [33] and Skindex-29 [34] and the 10 item Rosenberg Self-Esteem Scale [35].

In a recent study Bowe and colleagues looked at body image disturbance in patients with acne vulgaris. [36] 52 patients with acne attending an outpatient Dermatology clinic were assessed using validated questionnaires, including the Body Image Disturbance questionnaires (BIDQ) and objective physical grading of the severity of the subjects' acne. The general trend was that the more severe acne grade was associated with a greater psychosocial detriment, although patients who had mild acne still demonstrated emotional, social and behavioural impact, confirming that the severity of acne could not be predicted by any outsider without assessing these domains. The authors provide examples of written testimonials from subjects giving specific detail about the impact of acne on their lives. This has been shown in other informative qualitative studies from Koo [27] and Murray [29] . Therefore, it is the severity of the disease as perceived by the patient that is critical. As Dermatologists we hear such quotes from patients regularly, if we give them the time to talk and we actively listen.

Handstock and O'Mahony, examined the possible relationship between perfectionism, acne and appearance concerns in a group of 165 female University students. [37] Multiple regression analysis showed that after controlling for general psychopathology, a high level of socially prescribed perfectionism (i.e. the belief that others hold one to perfectionist standards and expectations) was associated with a greater tendency to be concerned about acne in particular and appearance in general. This adds to previous work suggesting that improvement in acne severity can reduce dysphoria (emotional pain) and lead to greater satisfaction with other unrelated body aspects, such as shape and weight. There has been much discussion and literature about the link between body image and acne. One theory is that people with acne become used to thinking about their appearance in a critical, negative and self-conscious manner and even when their acne subsides, these negative thoughts may remain. It is suggested that in susceptible individuals this may lead to Body Dysmorphic Disorder (BDD), which has its onset usually in adolescence, and often acne can be the trigger. [26] The term, "dysmorphic concern" has been suggested to describe the milder end of the BDD spectrum. [38] Indeed, this spectrum likely overlaps into what would be considered normal concern about appearance, particularly in adolescence. Other terms that Dermatologists may use include; "body image concern", "body image stress" or "acne dysmorphia". Handstock's findings showed a relation between acne related quality of life, body image concern and socially prescribed perfection. This latter characteristic was considered to be maladaptive and is an example of a negative self-schema. Participants who had greater severity facial acne in the past had greater current image concern. It is postulated that in susceptible individuals, even mild acne in adolescence may cause the person to place more importance on physical attractiveness in the future and tend to think of their appearance in a critical and negative way.

Cosmetic camouflage may have a role as a coping mechanism so boys at are at a disadvantage. The use of cosmetic camouflage may also be helpful in patients who have acne scarring as well as in active acne during the time between treatment initiation and visible beneficial effects. Corrective camouflage use was reported in a case series of 15 children and adolescents (age range, 7-16 years; mean age, 14 years). The majority of patients were girls. Six patients had acne vulgaris. The authors conclude that expert training from nurses in how to apply cosmetics may result in patient satisfaction, boosting self esteem and result in better psychosocial sequelae [39].

Hayashi et al. studied the effect of make-up use on quality of life in a small group of patients with acne [40] 18 female acne patients aged 13 – 38 years received lectures and practical training from a professional make-up artist on how to use make-up to conceal eruptions, e.g. to use complementary colours to camouflage eruptions and how to create a focal point to make the acne less obvious. Make-up was provided by a Japanese company specifically designed for people with acne and patients were treated with oral and/or topical antibiotics and chemical peeling along with the application of make-up for 2 to 4 weeks. Although not highly statistically significant, the results showed a trend towards less perceived acne severity –

- Number of inflammatory acne eruptions decreased from 10.0 to 6.5 ($P<0.01$)
- Non-inflammatory eruptions decreased from 15.1 to 10.1 ($P< 0.01$
- Leeds grading of global acne decreased from 4.3 to 3.3 ($P< 0.01$)
- Quality of life scores were taken before the make-up lessons and at the end point of the investigation using Skindex-16.
- Average symptom score decreased from 30.6 to 14.6 ($P<0.01$)
- Negative emotions decreased from 80 to 51 ($P<0.01$)

Appearance concern decreased from 89.2 to 63.5, frustration decreased from 83.3 to 46.9, embarrassment from 79.4 to 50.0, being annoyed from 89.6

to 63.5, feeling depressed from 79.4 to 52.1. Functional scores did not change significantly.

GHQ 30 score at baseline was > 9 before the make-up lessons but decreased to 5 after continuous make-up.

The average WHO QOL-26 showed slight improvement ($p<0.05$).

Depression-dejection, anger-hostility and fatigue of POMS (Profile of mood states) showed improvements also STAI (State-Trait Anxiety Inventory) revealed a prompt change of anxiety state after make-up lessons and that change remained until the end of this trial. Anxiety traits also improved.

Visual Analogue Scale (VAS) increased immediately after cosmetic lessons and remained improved (reduced but still statistically significant) at the end of the study demonstrating successful camouflage of the acne.

However, caution must be applied in interpreting these results in to clinical practice. The numbers were small and the study was sponsored by the manufacture of the "acne-friendly" make-up used. Also, the need for regular time-consuming thick make-up application may be maladaptive and may be associated with BDD.

A community based questionnaire study of 3775 18 year olds from Germany explored self-esteem and body satisfaction among late adolescents with acne. [41]

18 year olds were chosen because late adolescents (17-21) often make important life decisions e.g. long-term relationships, career choices, further education etc. It has been found in previous studies that during this final phase, integration of self-images and overall identity formation are dominant themes. It is thought that that high self-esteem is particularly significant in late adolescence, when major life choice are being made.

Experiencing high self-esteem may serve as a protective factor in coping with new and chronic illness, whereas low self-esteem is associated with anxiety, depression, and increased reports of general psychiatric symptoms.

The variables studied included –

- Depressive symptoms (Hopkins symptom checklist)
- Self-esteem (4 questions from Rosenburg self-esteem scale – self-attitude, uselessness, pride and self-worth)
- Body satisfaction/body image ("I am satisfied with my body". Options, strongly agree, agree, disagree, strongly disagree)
- Acne ("Have you had in the last week?": "Have you had any pimples?" – No, Yes a little, quite a lot or very much)
- Body mass index

Results

- Girls with acne had significantly higher levels of depressive symptoms than girls without (51% vs 32%)
- Girls with acne had significantly lower self-attitude than girls without (25% vs 16%)
- Girls with acne feel more useless than girls without (50% vs 36%)
- Girls with acne have lower self-worth than girls without (21% vs 11%)
- Girls with acne had poorer body satisfaction than girls without (56% vs 40%)
- Boys with acne had significantly higher levels of depressive symptoms compared to boys without acne (20% vs 14%)
- Boys with acne had lower self-attitude compared to boys without acne (13% vs 7%)
- Boys with acne had higher feeling of uselessness compared to boys without acne (29% vs 21%)
- Boys with acne had lower sense of pride compared to boys without acne (23% vs 16%)
- Boys with acne had lower self-worth compared to boys without acne (11% vs 7%)
- Boys with acne had poorer body satisfaction compared to boys without acne (27% vs 17%)

In all models depressive symptoms were significantly associated with serlf-esteem items and poor body satisfaction for both sexes where as BMI did not show any association.

For both sexes, acne could explain a low sense of pride and poor body image independently of BMI and depressive symptoms. Only boys showed lower self-attitude because of acne and only girls showed lower self-worth because of acne.

Quality of Life (Table 3)

Overall, considerable disability can be caused by acne as shown in some excellent research by Motley and Finlay, who subsequently devised a simple questionnaire to help quantify the degree of disability – the Cardiff Acne Disability Index. [13, 14]

A study by Cunliffe in 1986 found significantly higher levels of unemployment in patients with acne, compared to controls. [42] Previous research and clinical experience shows clearly that acne severity does not always correlate with patients' quality of life; some individuals suffer from severe acne with it having little effect on their lives, whereas in others, very mild acne can significantly impair the patient's life. This was demonstrated in a recent study of 112 female students attending a dermatology clinic with acne. [43] The Global Acne Grading System (GAGS) and Cardiff Acne Disability Index (CADI) were completed by physician. 82 cases were mild, 28 cases were moderate and 2 cases were severe. No correlation was found between CADI and GAGS. No correlation was found between CADI and the age of patients. No correlation was found between CADI and disease duration.

These results are consistent with findings in other studies looking at polpulations in several countries and reaffirms a potential lack of correlation between objective acne severity, quality of life, age and disease duration. Therefore there may be other reasons affecting the quality of life of acne patients other that acne severity. These other factors likely include social and emotional variables, personality type, presence of scarring and school/job related problems.

It is important not to overlook the patient's perspective in assessing acne severity.

Table 3. Potential adverse effects of acne on Quality of Life

local or systemic side-effects of topical or systemic treatment
time taken to apply treatment or make-up
interference socially eg. dating, eating out, relationship problems with partner, friends or relatives,
teasing, name-calling / bullying related to acne
sexual difficulties
interference with shopping, home-keeping or gardening
negative influence on choice of clothes
interference at school, college or work – impaired performance / avoidance / unemployment
interference with sports / hobbies eg. avoidance of swimming or shared changing facilities

A recent study from Turkey evaluated the correlation between quality of life scales and both the physician's and patient's assessments of acne severity. [44] 20 acne patients attending an outpatient clinic completed a simple 3-item questionnaire answered using a 10 point scale –

1. How much are you disturbed by your acne?
2. How severe do you think your acne is?
3. How much does oiliness of your skin disturb you?

The Turkish Acne Quality of Life (AQOL) form was completed – 9 questions. 50 patients also completed Short Form 36 (SF-36) a generic general health questionnaire measuring 8 dimensions of health

Patients were assessed by a Dermatologist using Global Acne Grading System (GAGS) and 27% - Mild, 54% - Moderate, 19% - Severe acne was found. There was no correlation found between the GAGS scores and any of the patient's own assessments.

The mean AQOL was 13.5. There was NO correlation between scores of GAGS and AQOL.

The AQOL correlated with the patient's own assessment for disturbance due to acne, acne severity and for disturbance due to oiliness

The AQOL correlated with the subgroups of SF-36 including social functioning, mental health and role limitations due to physical problems.

However the was no correlation between AQOL and subgroups of physical functioning, role limitations due to emotional problems, energy/vitality, pain and general health perceptions. There was no correlation between the subgroups of SF-36 and either GAGS or patient's own perceptions.

In one study, quality of life questionnaires were given to both children with skin diseases and children with other chronic physical diseases; acne patients scored almost as poorly as those with diabetes and epilepsy highlighting the huge impact of acne on a child's life. [45] In a similar study, adults with acne scored the impact of their disease on their quality of life as highly as those with asthma, epilepsy, chronic pain and diabetes [2] and it has also been shown that patients with acne, psoriasis and atopic eczema are more likely to pay for treatment of their disease than asthma, angina and hypertension patients [46].

Stress Exacerbating Acne

Stress and emotional factors have long been thought to influence the course of several skin diseases including acne. [47] The inflammatory component of acne is influenced by immunological factors. There is now convincing evidence that stress, both acute and chronic, influences the immune system, and therefore the fact that some patients with acne report deterioration in times of stress, should not come as a surprise. There are many sources of stress eg. sleep deprivation, school-related concerns, relationship problems. Adolescents report flare ups before social events or around exam times [2]. Stress may affect the pathophysiology of acne at several levels e.g. the hypothalamic-pituitary-adrenal axis, the production of vasoactive neuropeptides and humoral inflammatory mediators [48].

Sebaceous gland activity is under endocrine control and corticosteroids and adrenal androgens are produced in times of stress; this may result in increased seborrhoea and therefore worsen acne. [2] Recently, further scientific studies have added more weight to the stress-emotion hypothesis for acne. [49] The Neuro-Immuno-Cutaneous-Endocrine (N.I.C.E) model [50] is now accepted with stress-induced mediators having a negative impact on immune system functioning and increasing inflammatory mediators which may exacerbate the patient's acne worsening the secondary psychological impact of the disease. This "vicious circle" of skin disease maintenance [26] is seen commonly in other dermatoses eg. eczema and psoriasis with an accepted psychosomatic basis. Such stress-responders may benefit from relaxation training and other aspects of stress management. [8]

Secondary Emotional and Psychological Factors

Some people see their acne as a right of passage (as do some family doctors), however, others can suffer from severe psychological dysfunction in response to their condition, irrespective of the objective severity of disease. Some well-recognised psychological responses seen in acne patients include depressive symptoms, low self-esteem, social withdrawal, lack of confidence and even suicidal ideation and suicide attempts [2, 51, 52, 53] These psychological sequelae can, in turn, result in social, schooling, vocational, interpersonal, relationship and anger problems [54].

The psychological impact of acne vulgaris on patients' lives is often overlooked and underestimated by physicians. [2, 16] It seems illogical that the psychological effects of acne are not taken into consideration routinely: acne is rarely associated with systemic illness and is not a physically debilitating condition; therefore, the main reason for patient presentation is due to the cosmetic aversion of the disease. Patients often feel 'ugly' due to the effect acne has had on their appearance and makes them feel self-conscious. Facial appearance and body image have an important role to play in self-esteem, and self-esteem is a key influence in general psychological health [2, 42]. Therefore, a natural link between acne and psychosocial dysfunction is to be expected, in fact, studies have shown adult dermatological out patients have a 30- 40% prevalence of a psychiatric co-morbidity[15] and as many as 50% of 12-20 year olds with acne show negative psychological responses to their disease [17]. However, most patients with acne do not have severe associated psychological morbidity and one needs to avoid "psychologicalising" such individuals unnecessarily.

There is a spectrum of emotional sequelae secondary to acne: some individuals appear to be extremely stoical and resistant to emotional morbidity with positive coping mechanisms, even with objectively severe acne on physical examination; other individuals appear to be more prone to emotional morbidity even when objectively there is mild acne; the reasons for this are complex and have been addressed in several studies. Maladaptive coping can manifest as a variety of behaviours (Table 4).

Table 4. Potential maladaptive behavioural coping mechanisms associated with acne

Excessive use of commercial tanning salons
repeated mirror-checking / mirror avoidance
use of clothing or body to cover affected areas
excessive touching or interfering with affected areas
compulsive picking or squeezing of affected areas
long-term use of heavy make-up
excessive alcohol or recreational drug use
excessive ritualistic cleansing regimens
repeated reassure seeking
repeated internet-searches for "miracle cure"
repeated purchase of "miracle" acne products
regular comparison with others, photographs in magazines, TV or film actors/actresses
avoidance of social events

Table 5. Potential psychiatric Disorders associated with Acne

adjustment disorder
depressive disorder
social phobia and anxiety disorder
eating disorder
obsessive-compulsive disorder
Body Dysmorphic Disorder

When such behaviours are extreme, an associated psychiatric disorder should be considered (table 5)

Illness Perception – Myths and Misconceptions

Exploring the patients perceived ideas and illness perception is useful as it may uncover unhelpful errors in thinking with associated negative feelings and unhelpful actions eg. someone may feel that acne is caused by being unclean and so think that other people consider them to be dirty and as a result clean their skin many times a day and try to squeeze out the "germs". These areas can be discussed and the patient guided as appropriate. An important component in patient management is patient education at the time of the initial consultation [2]. It has been found that both patients and the general public have a poor understanding of what causes acne and that many think that personal hygiene plays a big role; thus resulting in the purchase of over-the-counter creams and face-washes, which can, in fact, worsen the acne and delay presentation to health professionals [2]. Therefore, it is important to explore the patient's understanding, fears and expectations in regard to their acne. Educating the patient may allow them to avoid products and activities, such as excessive face washing, which can worsen their acne. The doctor may also be able to dispel preconceived ideas about acne and ameliorate some of their negative ruminations regarding their skin condition. In fact one paper states: "A lack of proper education about acne can feed into the negativity associated with the disease and foster an environment of depression and anxiety" [55].

Patient education not only involves explaining the aetiology of the condition and the avoidance of factors that may make it worse, it also includes education about treatment and psychoeducation to help the person understand their thoughts, feelings and behaviours related to acne.

Table 6. Potential resilience factors aiding coping with acne

Preacne positive personality factors
Optimum psychological well-being
Self-determining and independent, self-efficacy
Self-acceptance – positive attitude toward self, accepts good and bad qualities both physical and emotional, feels positive about past life, high self-esteem, self-mastery
optimism
Peer popularity
Leadership qualities
Sporting high achiever
Strong family bonding and warm, trusting relationships with others
Stable family dynamics
Good at emotional disclosure
Use of humour
"thick skinned" to adverse comments

Education is not synonymous with understanding and one must be wary of information over-load but rather give small "chunks" at a time which the person can digest and then apply to themselves. Adherence to medical treatment has been shown to be poor in the general population and perhaps even poorer in adolescence. Motivational interviewing may help in this regard. One must be aware that in some adolescents, their acne may be used as an excuse for refusing to go to school or take part in activities due to an already unstable emotional status. [19]

Positive Coping Factors and Resilience versus Risks Factors for Impaired Coping

A person may have objectively mild severity acne but which has a huge impact on their quality of life. Conversely we see some adolescents with physically severe, inflammatory acne that appear to be coping extremely well, with minimal secondary disability. These people appear to have resilience factors which may include popularity at school, attractive physical attributes or sporting ability. (Table 6)

Panconesi has suggested that such youngsters have charisma and leadership qualities which contribute towards self esteem [56].

In recent years there has been much research and commentary on the role of psychological well-being and the presence of resilience factors in coping with adverse life events including physical disease. [57] These factors can be both internal eg. character strengths and external in the form of family and friend support. The presence of such psychosocial resources can help buffer the effects of rising distress and help coping. As yet there is little research in this area with skin diseases including acne but one could postulate similar findings to that found with other chronic disease eg. diabetes mellitus. [58]

In contrast, lack of factors that can promote resilience and positive coping can be associated with risk for poor coping (Table 7).

A recent study examined the role of friendships and social acceptance in perceptions of appearance and emotional resilience in adolescents with and without a facial difference. [59] The emotional functioning in adolescents with cleft lip and palate was studied. The investigators postulated that positive social experiences counteract potential negative self-views of appearance, and consequently protect against depressive symptoms while negative social experiences would be thought to reinforce negative self-perceptions of appearance and exacerbate emotional distress.

289 16-year-olds attending the Oslo cleft lip and palate clinic participated (196 with visible cleft, 93 with a non-visible cleft)

A comparison group of 1832 adolescents was taken from a large national survey. Any depressive symptoms were recorded using the 6-item shortened version of Hopkins symptom checklist.

Friendship and social acceptance variables were also recorded - close friendships, social acceptance and self perceptions of physical appearance.

Compared to comparison group adolescents with a visible cleft reported:

- More positive perceptions of close friendships
- Higher levels of social acceptance
- More positive self-perceptions of appearance
- Less emotional distress

Only social acceptance differed significantly between the two groups of adolescents with a cleft. The most positive self-perceptions were reported by the adolescents with a visible difference. Surprisingly adolescents with a non-visible cleft were more satisfied with their appearance than the comparison group.

Table 7. Potential risk factors for maladaptive coping with acne

Personality factors – social sensitivity, low self esteem
"thin skinned" nature
Suboptimal or impaired psychological well-being
Social perfectionism – overconcerned with the expectations and evaluations of others, conforms to social pressures
Lack of self-acceptance - dissatisfaction with self, disappointed with what has occurred in past life, troubled by certain personal qualities – wishes to be different
Few close relationships with others, difficulty being open, feeling of isolation, lack of support from family and friends
Dysfunctional family dynamics
Early maladaptive schemas and ongoing negative self schemas (unhelpful expectations of other people's behaviour)

The main results revealed that adolescents with a visible difference reported better functioning on all study variables compare to the comparison group.

This study suggests that adolescents with a facial difference may have developed skills to cope with the consequences of the cleft. It was suggested that efforts are made by the affected individual and their families to strengthen positive aspects of friendships and social experiences, thus protecting the adolescents against the negative effects of facial difference.

This would suggest that it may be fruitful to strengthen close friendships and social acceptance as a way of preventing and treating appearance-related distress in children and adolescents that look different as in acne. It may be that people with a congenital disfigurement usually adjust better that those with an acquired disfigurement eg. acne. However, those people with objectively severe acne who do adjust and cope well may share similar innate attributes with those with a cleft palate.

Results from future research in this area will be very interesting.

4 Groups Meriting Special Consideration

1. Persistent Facial Acne in the Older Women

Women tend to get the short straw with regard to chronic acne especially in a perioral distribution. This can cause significant psychoemotional distress and the phenomenon of "learned helplessness" with pessimism and depressive symptoms may develop as described by Seligman [60].

All women in this subgroup merit a psychosomatic approach with treatment individualised as per clinical need. [61] Long-term low dose oral isotretinoin may be needed to achieve satisfactory control.

2. Acne Scarring

Scars, like other visible changes of skin, have a unique impact on patients' lives. In recent years there has been some pioneering research into the effect of scarring on people's quality of life from the McGrouther group based in Manchester, England. [62, 63, 64]

These authors report five main areas of impact on people with scars lives: physical comfort and functioning; acceptability to self and others; social functioning; confidence in the nature and management of the condition and emotional well-being. The majority of respondents were unhappy with their scar's appearance due to their perceived stigma and psychological associations, and thus adopted different coping behaviours to hide or compensate for them. Often this made them unsociable and interfered with their communication skills, personal relationships, work life and leisure activities. Concerns about the diagnosis and persistent nature of scars were common, whilst unempathic management by general physicians and frustrations of current treatment compounded distress.

Transcribed qualitative data underwent interpretative phenomenological analysis to identify common themes in individuals' personal experiences.

A scar-specific patient-reported outcome measure was developed and validated – "The Patient-Reported Impact of Scars Measure". [65] This assessment tool has two unidimensional scales with good psychometric and scaling properties. Reproducibility was adequate for the symptom scale consisting of 13 questions (0.83) and good for the quality-of-life scale consisting of 22 questions (0.89).

It is well accepted by patients and easy to use, and is useful for assessing scar disease severity in clinical practice.

As with acne, correlation between psychosocial distress and objective scar severity may not be found. Again, as for acne, there does tend to be a correlation between psychosocial distress and subjective severity as perceived by the patient. [66] Interestingly, patients with non-visible scars experienced greater psychosocial distress than patients with visible scars. Scar type was unrelated to psychosocial distress. Therefore patient self-assessment should form an integral part of clinical assessment of acne scars.

3. Acne Excoriee

Acne excoriee is a sub-type of acne vulgaris. Acneiform lesions are repeatedly manipulated often by picking or squeezing. Often the disorder runs a chronic course over many years and is resistant to conventional physical therapy. In an interesting paper from 1983, Sneddon and Sneddon suggest that the behaviour is "a protective device to conceal an emotional failure". [65] They report a case series of 8 patients all female who were treated with antipsychotic oral therapy and supportive psychotherapy. Minimal improvement was seen and "a phobic state was revealed that had been previously hidden from the patient". Some patients had no present evidence of active acne suggesting a diagnosis of neurotic excoriations. All patients had a history of neurotic symptoms since childhood on enquiry which the authors suggest may be contributive eg. social phobia, poor relationships with parents or partner, poor self-image, bed-wetting, difficulty sleeping, recurrent nightmares, nail biting, thumb sucking, stammer, school phobia, travel phobia, fear of vomiting. Another paper assessed 12 patients with acne excoriee and reported contrasting results with minimal associated psychopathology. [66] 2/12 exhibited dysthymia and 2/12 had a personality disorder. Most of the 12 patients reported a concern for being unattractive and a compulsive urge to manipulate their skin. However, 8/12 patients did not fulfill the criteria for a psychiatric disorder. There was no evidence of underlying obsessive-compulsive disorder or body image disorder. Therefore, it would appear that there may or may not be underlying primary or secondary psychopathology and stress may contribute to exacerbations. A combined therapeutic approach is optimal including psychological assessment, supportive psychotherapy, education, cognitive therapy when needed and behavioural therapy eg. habit reversal training. [67] Low dose, long-term oral isotretionoin may help. A therapeutic trial of an SSRI or antipsychotic agent can be used in stubborn cases. [68]

4. Acne Dysmorphia and Body Dysmorphic Disorder

Over the last 20 years or so there has been an increasing volume of literature on Body Dysmorphic Disorder (BDD). This disorder has specific diagnostic criteria and was described in 1987 as a distinct psychiatric diagnosis. Katherine Philips is a leader in research into BDD and her excellent book, "The Broken Mirror" discusses the condition in detail. [69] BDD is defined as "a distressing and impairing preoccupation with an imagined or minor physical defect in appearance". The symptoms cannot be explained by any other underlying psychiatric diagnosis e.g. anorexia nervosa or bulimia.

Essentially such patients have a grossly disproportionate concern of a physical attribute that they consider as ugly or disfiguring and this causes significant emotional distress and secondary behavioural modification. Such patients develop a morbid preoccupation with an essentially normal appearance or a minor blemish. BDD is relatively common – studies have shown about 1% prevalence in the general population. It is over-represented in dermatology patients as 65% of patients with BDD have a cutaneous concern especially acne. There is a range of severity of BDD but up to 1/5 patients with acne would screen positive [70] These patients often initially present to a dermatologist, with self-perceived severe acne being one of the most common concerns [71]. When acne appears to be the only concern one may use the term acne dysmorphia. These patients may be under-diagnosed but it is important for Dermatologists to recognise this strong association and tailor treatment accordingly. Screening methods can be used easily in clinical practice. The first tool is usually a simple visual analogue scale, comparing the patients perceived ugliness as opposed to a neutral observer's objective appearance about how obvious or disfiguring the apparent blemish is, which may be the severity of acne graded using a validated objective scoring. When there is a discrepancy of > 5 in the 10 point scale, this is deemed to be disproportionate concern and would therefore lead to further assessment eg use of the Body Dysmorphic Disorder Modification of the Yale-Brown Obsessive-Compulsive Scale (Y-BOCS). [72]

In severe cases where there is the unshakable belief, help from liaison Psychiatry in the form of a joint consultation is desirable. Use of Roaccutane in such patients has been shown to be effective but relapse is common unless accompanied with associated psychological therapy using a cognitive behavioural approach. [73] A review of Cognitive Behavioural Therapy (CBT) for BDD is described by one of the experts in the field, David Veale. [74] Engagement is key with the development of a trusting, non-judgemental, therapeutic relationship. Self-help in the form of bibliotherapy [71] can aid progress. Referral for help from colleagues in mental health is desirable in more severely affected individuals exhibiting significant clinical depression, social withdrawal and occupational impairment secondary to BDD – such patients have a significant risk of suicide as reported by Cotterill and Cunliffe in 1997, and so this group of patients must not be underestimated [52]. Dermatologists should be able to perform a basic assessment for suicidal risk to identify the high risk patient and when to seek urgent psychiatric assistance. [75] (See Table 8).

Table 8. Risk Factors for Suicide by a patient with acne

Large emotional impact Large psychological impact Large effect on quality of life Maladaptive coping mechanisms	situation felt to be causing unbearable distress
Absence of resilience factors Presence of risk factors for impaired coping Known psychiatric co-morbidity Body Dysmorphic Disorder Previous deliberate self-harm / overdose Thoughts of death Suicidal fantasies or ideation – not easily dismissed Family history of suicide Specific plans with access to potentially lethal means significant drug or alcohol use	signs suggestive of current mental illness

More Detailed Psychological Assessment and the Role of Psychometric Testing with Validated Questionnaires

It is best practice to assess patients who have acne for associated psychological comorbidities to achieve maximum benefit and minimise risk to the patient. The use of validated general health questionnaires, mental health questionnaires and dermatology-specific and acne-specific questionnaires can also help in information gathering and is particularly important to a dermatologist without experience in mental health. When psychiatric comorbidity is present, it should be addressed and treated and when necessary, referral to a specialist in mental health is desirable. Simple measures like use of SUbjective Discomfort Scores (SUDS) self-reported by the patient, assessing general well-being, anxiety, depression and stress are a good starting point and when low scores are obtained, this may be reassuring and suggests a "low risk" patient in whom conventional dermatological treatment is likely to suffice. [8] In recent years guidelines have suggested routine screening for depression in adults with various chronic diseases. It is known that chronic disease is a risk factor for depressive symptoms, including clinical depression, so this would seem logical. However, it is perhaps not as simple as it may seem, and there is the potential for various pitfalls when this is performed by non-experts in Mental Health. [76] There is a high prevalence of psychiatric morbidity in the general population (about 30%) and this may be slightly higher in adult dermatology patients (up to 40%). [20] This morbidity may go unrecognised and so untreated, which could result in adverse consequences. Various screening tools can help to identify symptoms that may suggest depression in patients. In an excellent paper by Hinkle and colleagues, four commonly used questionnaires were assessed in terms of their sensitivity and specificity and ease of use. [77] The authors concluded that the World Health Organisation - 5 Wellbeing Index performed best. This can be used as the first part of a 2 part screening process for depression in acne patients. It is a simple 5 statement self-assessment form referring to the person's feeling over the previous 2 weeks. There are 5 statements and the answer to which is graded from 'all the time' scoring 5 points to 'no time' scoring nil points. The 5 statements are:

1. I felt cheerful and in good spirits
2. I have felt calm and relaxed
3. I have felt active and vigorous
4. I woke up feeling fresh and rested
5. My day life has been filled with things that interest me

Total scores calculated by adding the figures of the 5 answers, with zero representing the worst possible score and 25 the best possible wellbeing score. It is advised that if the score is below 13, further more detailed assessment is desirable. The score can be used in monitoring change with 10% difference indicating significant change.

Previous studies have shown that Dermatologists underestimate the prevalence of psychiatric disorders. [16] General Practitioners also may under diagnose a depressive disorder. [76] There is a concern amongst Dermatologists that there could be a risk of over diagnosing psychiatric disorder and labelling a patient inappropriately. Therefore it can be helpful to enquire about wellbeing rather than symptoms of depression. There are 9 cardinal symptoms of depressive disorder – 5 mental (low mood, lack of interest or enjoyment in usual activities, decreased concentration, guilty thoughts, suicidal thoughts) and 4 physical (sleep disturbance either hypersomnulence or insomnia, appetite disturbance either increased or decreased, decreased energy or restless excessive energy, psychomotor slowing or agitation). [78] Generating a list of symptoms can be helpful – 5/9 cardinal symptoms may indicate depressive disorder. One must recognise the limitations of such an approach as compared to a semi-structured psychiatric interview performed by a specialist. It also must be stated that a positive screening does not necessarily represent a diagnosis of depression, risk of depression or a need for any treatment.[75] However, it does give some useful information that can be used for future comparison, especially if the patient is on a medication that may adversely affect mood e.g. oral Isotretinoin. The Hospital Anxiety and Depression Scale (HADS) is one of many validated depression screening questionnaires that may be used to help in assessment of the presence and severity of symptoms. [79]

Assessment of the Psychological Impact of Acne

At present there is not a universally accepted assessment tool for measuring quality of life and the psychosocial impact of acne. More than 10 different questionnaires/assessment tools have been used [80]. This makes it very difficult to compare data from different studies.

It must also be considered that acne may not be the only thing affecting quality of life. The patient may, for example, have difficult social circumstances, other medical problems or pre-existing psychological disorders and not all of the screening tools used take this in to account, are specific enough in their wording or are even specific to acne.

DLQI [33] is the tool most used in the UK but its efficacy has been challenged recently. [81] Only 1 of the 10 questions addresses emotional morbidity asking, "how embarrassed or self-conscious have you been because of your skin?" The other 9 questions ask about physical symptoms, daily activities, leisure, work and school, personal relationships and treatment-related mess or time. In contrast, Skindex-29 has 29 items arranged in 3 scales (7 symptoms, 10 emotions and 12 functioning) and so it is more comprehensive. DLQI and Skindex have been compared recently. [82]

Ideally, a standardised disease specific tool could be devised that can be used globally for all acne patients. Such a tool should be both sensitive and specific in capturing changes in acne severity relating to impact on all aspects of quality of life. This would provide useful information to the practitioner and be useful for data analysis. However, to date this had not been possible due to various confounding factors related to age group and sex as it is known that depression and anxiety are more common in women than men [16] and that clinically diagnosed depression has been shown to be higher in older acne patients [5, 17, 55]. This screening tool could then, perhaps, highlight 'red flags' that may help in recognising patients that are suffering from negative psychological impact due to their disease and this could then be explored further by the practitioner. A generic quality of life or depression screening tool is still useful in highlighting a patient that is already struggling with poor quality of life or depression. Any screening tool results, however, need to be correctly interpreted by the doctor, who can then spend more time in their initial and further consultations exploring the patients hopes, fears and expectations of their disease and treatment and to give them extra support to potentially avoid excessive negative psychosocial impact of their acne on their life.

Extending the examination from being poorly dermatological to assessing areas that reflect the patients' underlying psyche is essential to identify patients at risk. There are 10 components of a mental status examination [78]-

1. Appearance and general behaviour
2. Motor activity
3. Speech
4. Mood and affect
5. Thought process
6. Thought content
7. Perceptual disturbances
8. Sensorium and cognition
9. Insight
10. Judgement

A full structured psychiatric assessment of mental status is outwith the ability of most Dermatologists to perform and interpret but with observation of patients' behaviour, obvious or more subtle signs can be detected. Thus a psychologically-minded dermatologist can, with experience and effort, fine-tune his psychological "radar" and develop an ability to detect verbal and non-verbal 'red flag' signs. [3] However, it would appear that the detection of patients' psychoemotional morbidity by many dermatologists is not completely satisfactory and the signs are missed due to the apparent presence of psychological "scotoma" [16] Warning signs in the patients' general behaviour include: withdrawn, guarded, hostile, irritable, resistant, very shy or defensive nature. Other alarm bells include, fleeting, sporadic or avoided eye contact.

A well groomed immaculate appearance may suggest perfectionism or obsessive compulsive nature.

Thick make-up may suggest underlying impairment of self image which can be associated with acne dysmorphia or body dysmorphic disorder.

An unkempt appearance may suggest self neglect which can be associated with depressive disorder.

Paranoid or delusional patients may have a very guarded manner.

Paucity of speech can be associated with depressive disorder.

Obvious tremor, restlessness and sweating can be found with anxiety disorder. Repeated angry and negative comments, which can contribute towards a "difficult" consultation, have been shown to be associated with underlying psychopathology and in adolescents may represent an expression of depressive symptoms [3] Observed compulsive behaviours in the consultation, including picking at the skin may suggest a compulsive disorder.

Shared intense feelings of melancholia, agitation, anger and irritability and suicidal ideation are particularly significant and may warrant formal psychiatric assessment. Further enquiry regarding thought content may reveal unorthodox fixed beliefs, obsessions, phobias and frank delusions, again which would warrant further formal psychiatric assessment.

Thus, a pre-assessment screening tool plus a list of criteria for the doctor to be aware of in consultation could possibly pick up those patients who are at high risk of not coping well and extra support or referral to mental health professionals could be offered. Suicide risk should be assessed when needed (Table 8).

Psychopharmaceutical therapy can be initiated when indicated either by the psychologically-minded dermatologist, the patient's General Practitioner or a psychiatrist.

Oral Isotretinoin as a Psychotropic Drug – What Is the Evidence for Increased Suicidality?

There has been much written about the possible association between oral Isotretinoin and depression and suicide since the original reporting came to light in 2000. In summary, between 1982 and 2000 the food and drug administration (FDA) received reports of 431 cases of depression, suicidal ideation, suicide attempts or suicide in US patients treated with Isotretinoin. [83] There were 37 patients who committed suicide, 24 of them while using Isotretinoin, 13 after ceasing to use it. A history of psychiatric illness was reported for 8/37 patients (22%). Median peak dose was 1mg/kg body weight. During the same period the FDA analysed reports of 110 American patients who were hospitalised for depression while using Isotretinoin (85 patients) or after stopping its use (25 patients). The median time of use of the drug before hospitalisation was 1 month. For those who had stopped using it, the median interval in stopping use in hospitalisation was 3 months. A history of psychiatric illness was reported for 48 of these patients (44%). In many patients there was improvement after discontinuation of the drug and psychiatric treatment, but others had persistent depression after the drug was discontinued. 4 patients were re-challenged with Isotretinoin; symptoms developed again in 1 and the other 3 were able to continue using the drug at a reduced dose. It must be stated that the number of suicide reports among users of Isotretinoin did not exceed the number that would be predicted on the basis of the suicide rate in the USA. However, Isotretinoin was in the top 10 drugs in the FDA's database in terms of the number of reports of depression and suicidal attempts among its users. The possible explanation for the high number of such reports are better reporting than for other drugs and the confounding factor of a relation between acne and depressive symptoms. Since this data came to light, many investigators have tried to clarify the matter. Kellett and Gawkrodger in 2005 reported the result of a prospective study of the responsiveness of depression and suicidal ideation in acne patients to different phases of Isotretinoin therapy. [84] Depressive symptoms and quality of life improved universally. However, isolated case reports of adverse mental health outcomes in patients taking roaccutane continue. In an excellent comprehensive review recently published, Bremner and colleagues scrutinised the evidence for an association between retinoic acid and affective disorders in great detail. [85] They examined the data on the neuropsychiatric effects of vitamin A, look at individual case reports of depressive symptoms following Isotretinoin treatment and surmise evidence of an association from group studies and larger database studies. There is considerable evidence that Isotretinoin, when used for acne, has positive behavioural effects with improved self-image and quality of life, but this is not the same as curing clinical depression, and they argue the case that acne has not been proven to be causative of clinical depression. Temporary relationship between the Isotretinoin treatment and exacerbation of pre-existing clinical depression or depressive symptoms is convincing, although appears to be rare. There is some evidence for a dose response effect for Isotretinoin and psychiatric side effects, with high doses associated with more side effects. There certainly is considerable biological plausibility that Isotretinoin in psychotropic. An interesting theoretical study that would be very useful to clarity this complex topic would be a double blinded placebo-controlled randomised trial assessing the effects of Isotretinoin on symptoms of depression and mood lability, but it was felt it would be too difficult adequately blind because of the ubiquitous dry skin side effects of Isotretinoin. These authors conclude that based on the literature to date, Dermatologists should be very cautious as to whether to re-challenge patients who have previous experience depressive symptoms whilst taking Isotretinoin. The treatment of patients with known psychiatric disorders, especially bipolar disorder, appears to pose a higher risk for exacerbation of symptoms and consultation with colleagues in Mental Health is recommended in such cases. It is the authorss' opinion that treatment with oral isotretinoin is relatively indicated in all patients with acne of any objective severity (including acne dysmorphia) who have significant psychoemotional morbidity with associated large impact on quality of life. However, there is a wide range of therapeutic timidity in using roaccutane in patients with low mood or history of psychiatric disorder and other dermatologists have a higher threshold for roaccutane use in such groups. It should be emphasised that withholding roaccutane can be as harmful or more harmful than giving roaccuatane. Although the vast majority of people taking Isotretinoin for acne will not have any significant adverse psychiatric side effects, there is a small at risk group, and so it is important to discuss openly the possible side effects with each patient and reduce the dose or stop Roaccutane when necessary.

Discussion

It would be useful to routinely classify every person with acne in terms of objective physical severity and impact on quality of life. In those with minimal impact on quality of life who are psychologically stable, conventional dermatological treatment will likely suffice. In those with a large impact on quality of life a psychosomatic approach is optimum using both physical and psychological therapy. A large impact on quality of life may be associated with significant psychopathology. Further assessment for specific psychiatric disorder is then desirable. Acne does represent a paradigm of a biopsychosocial disease which is influenced by many factors, resulting in either a balance or imbalance and therefore coping or impaired coping. Therefore, an extended examination of the acne patient is desirable to include the impact on quality of life, as well as the presence or absence of psychological and emotional factors, to allow holistic approach and optimise the chance of improvement in all variables. A biopsychosocial approach to the acne patient is the gold-standard approach. It involves integrating aspects of the traditional medical model of care with aspects of the educational and psychological models of care. It is possible that it is not used more often in practice due to lack of training, lack of confidence and lack of time in clinic. Also, as acne is a clear and common diagnosis with a recognised medical model of care with recognised physical treatments, some doctors may believe this is adequate.

Conclusion

Objective acne clinical severity alone does not predict quality of life. The detrimental effect of acne on a person's quality of life forms a spectrum of severity from withdrawal tendencies to active suicidal ideation. This effect can be graded using validated quality of life assessment questionnaires.

Quality of life and depression assessment tools have been found to be useful for identifying these patients, but as of yet there is no uniform screening tool that is both thorough enough and specific enough to acne. Therefore, the use of several assessment tools may help capture a wider range of important psychoemotional and social variables. Efforts should be made to allow for more time for individual patients who have unmet needs, and a multidisciplinary approach using perhaps an experienced nurse to listen to, and talk with appropriate patients in a counselling capacity or indeed referral to colleagues in Clinical Psychology or liaison Psychiatry when necessary. A motivated, trained and knowledgeable Dermatologist can help patients who have acne and significant psychosocial detriment with a well thought out, planned, holistic approach using conventional topical therapy, oral therapy, including isotretinoin, and psychological therapy whether it be supportive, motivational or cognitive-behavioural and occasionally psychopharmacological therapy. This psychosomatic approach will result in better patient outcomes with increased patient satisfaction.

References

[1] Sulzberger MB, Zaidens SH. Psychogenic factors in dermatologic disorders. *Med. Clin. North Am.* 1948 May;32:669-85.

[2] V Niemeier, J Kupfer,U Gieler. Acne vulgaris – Psychosomatic aspects. *J. Dtsch. Dermatol. Ges.* 2006; 4(12):1027-36.
[3] R G fried, A Wechsler. Psychological problems in the acne patient. *Dermatol. Ther.* 2006; 19(4);237-40. 4.
[4] Koblenzer C. Psychosomatic Concepts in Dermatology. *Arch. Dermatol.* 1983; 501-512.
[5] J N Newton, E Mallon, A Klassen. The effectiveness of acne treatment: an assessment by patients of the outcome of therapy. *Br. J. Dermatol.* 1997; 137:563-7.
[6] Yentzer B, Gosnell A, Clark A, Pearce D et al. A randomised controlled pilot study of strategies to increase adherence in teenagers with acne vulgaris. *J. Am. Acad. Dermatol.* 2011; 64: 793-795.
[7] Koblenzer C. Psychotherapy for intractable inflammatory dermatoses. *Journal of the American Academy of Dermatology*. 1995;32:609-12.
[8] Shenefelt P. Psychodermatological disorders: recognition and treatment. *Int. Journ. Dermatol.* 2011; 50: 1309-1322.
[9] Obermayer ME. *Psychocutaneous Medicine* 1955, Thomas.
[10] Kenyon. FE. Psychosomatic aspects of acne: A controlled study. *Trans. St John's Hosp. Dem. Soc.* 1966;52:71-8.
[11] Maddin S. Current Concepts in the Management of Acne Vulgaris. *Canad. Med. Ass. J.* Feb. 15, 1969, vol. 100. 340-343.
[12] Shuster S. The effect of skin disease on self image. *Br. J. Dermatol.* 1978;99 (suppl 16): 18-19.
[13] Motley R, Finlay AY. How much disability is caused by acne? *Clinical and Experimental Dermatology*. 1989; 14: 194-198.
[14] Motley R, Finlay AY. Practical use of a disability index in the routine management of acne. *Clinical and Experimental Dermatology*. 1992; 17:1-3.
[15] Fava GA. Psychosomatic medicine. *Int. J. Clin. Pract.* July 2010; 64: 1155-1161.
[16] A Picardi, D Abenti, C F Melchi, P Puddu, P Pasquini. Psychiatric morbidity in dermatological outpatients: an issue to be recognized. *Br. J. Dermatology* 2000; 143(5):983-91.
[17] A Smithard, C Glazebrooke, H C Williams. Acne prevalence, knowledge about acne and psychological morbidity in mid-adolescence: a community-based study. *Br. J. Dermatology* 2001; 145(2): 274-9.
[18] Koblenzer CS. *Psychocutaneous Disease*. 1987, Grune and Stratton, Inc.

[19] Poot F. Doctor-patient relations in dermatology: obligations and rights for a mutual satisfaction. *J. Eur. Acad. Dermatol. Venereol.* 2009 Nov;23(11):1233-9.
[20] Harth W, Gieler U, Kusnir D, Tausk F. *Clinical Management in Psychodermatology*. 2009, Springer.
[21] Dorland's Medical Dictionary for Health Consumers. © 2007 by Saunders, an imprint of Elsevier, Inc.
[22] McGraw-Hill Concise Dictionary of Modern Medicine. © 2002 by The McGraw-Hill Companies, Inc.
[23] Ritvo E et al. Psychosocial judgements and perceptions of adolescents with acne vulgaris: A blinded, controlled comparison of adult and peer evaluations. *BioPsychoSocial Medicine* 2011, 5:11.
[24] Roosta N *et al*. Skin disease and stigma in emerging adulthood: impact on health development. *J. Cut. Med. Surg.* 2010; 14:285-90.
[25] Lowe JG. The stigma of acne. *Br. J. Hosp. Med.* 1993 Jun 2-15;49(11):809-12.
[26] Kellett S, Gilbert B. Acne: A biopsychosocial and evolutionary perspective with a focus on shame. *British Journal of health Psychology.* 2001; 6: 1-24.
[27] Koo J. The psychosocial impact of acne: patients' perceptions. *J. Am. Acad. Dermatol.* 1995; 32:S26-30.
[28] Gupta MA, Gupta AK. The psychological comorbidity in acne. *Clin. Dermatol.* 2001; 19:360-3.
[29] Murray CD, Rhodes K. 'Nobody likes damaged goods': The experience of adult visible acne. *British Journal of Health Psychology.* 2005;10:183-202.
[30] Medansky RS, Handler EM, Medansky DL. Self-evaluation of acne and emotion: A pilot study. *Psychosomatics* 1981;22:379-83.
[31] Krejci-Manwaring J. et al. Social sensitivity and acne: the role of personality in negative social consequences and quality of life. Int. J. Psychiatry Med. 2006; 36:121-30.
[32] Cash, T F and Pruzinsky T, Editors. Body Image Handbook of Theory Research in Clinical Practice, NY, Guildford Press (2002).
[33] Finlay AY, Khan GK. Dermatology Life Quality Index (DLQI) – a simple practical measure for routine clinical use. *Clin. Exp. Dermatol.* 1994:19:210-16.
[34] Chren MM, Lasek RJ, Flocke SA, Zyzanski SJ. Improved discriminative and evaluative capability of a refined version of Skindex, a quality of

life instrument for parients with skin diseases. *Arch. Dermatol.* 1997; 133: 1433-1440.
[35] Tinakon W, Nahathai W. A Comparison of Reliability and Construct Validity between the Original and Revised Versions of the Rosenberg Self-Esteem Scale. *Psychiatry Investig.* 2012 Mar;9(1):54-8. Epub 2012 Jan 25.
[36] Bowe W. et al. Body Image Disturbance in Patients with Acne Vulgaris. *The Journal of Clinical Aesthetic Dermatology.* 2011; 4: 35-41.
[37] Hanstock T, O'Mahony J. Perfectionism, acne and appearance concerns. *Personality and Individual Differences.* 2002; 32: 1317-1325.
[38] Phillips KA. Body Dysmorphic disorder and cosmetic dermatology: more than skin deep. *J. Cosmet. Dermatol.* 2004; 3:99-103.
[39] Tedeschi A, Dall'Oglio F, Micali G, Schwartz RA, Janniger CK. Corrective camouflage in pediatric dermatology. *Cutis.* 2007 Feb;79(2):110-2.
[40] Nobukazu Hayashi, Mizuho Imori, Midori Yanagisawa, Yoko Seto, Makoto Kawashima. Make-up improves the quality of life of acne patients without aggravating acne eruptions during treatments. *Eur. J. Dermatology* 2005; 15 (4): 284-7.
[41] Florence Dalgard, Uwe Gieler, Jan Oivind Holm, Espen Bjertness, Stuart Hauser. Self-esteem and body satisfaction among late adolescents with acne: Results from a population survey. *J. Am. Academy of Dermatology* 2008; 59: 743-751.
[42] Cunliffe WJ. Acne and unemployment. *Br. J. Dermatol.* 1986 Sep;115(3):386.
[43] Kokandi A. Evaluation of Acne Quality of Life and Clinical Severity in Acne Female Adults. *Dermatology Research and Practice* 2010. pii: 410809. Epub 2010 Jul 27.
[44] Zeynep Demircay, Dilek Seckin, Asli Senol, Figen Demir, Patient's perspective: an important issue not to be overlooked in assessing acne severity. *European Journ. Dermatol.* 2008; 18 (2): 181-4.
[45] P E Beattie, M S Lewis-Jones. A comparative study of impairment of quality of life in children with skin disease and children with other chronic childhood diseases. *Br. J. Dermatology* 2006; 155(1):145-51.
[46] L Parks, R Balkrishnan, L Hamel-Gariépy, S R Feldman. The importance of skin disease as assessed by 'willingness- to-pay'. *J. Cut. Med. and Surg.* 2003; 7(5):369-71.
[47] Griesemer RD. Emotionally triggered disease in a dermatological practice. *Psychiatr. Ann.* 1978; 8: 49-56.

[48] Misery L Skin, immunity and the nervous system. *Br. J. Dermatol.* 1997 Dec; 137(6):843-50.
[49] Ganceviciene R, Graziene V, Fimmel S et al. (2009) Involvement of the corticotropin-releasing hormone system in the pathogenesis of acne vulgaris. *Br. J. Dermatol.* 160:345–52.
[50] O'Sullivan RL, Lipper G, Lerner EA. The neuroimmuno-cutaneous-endocrine network: relationship of mind and skin. *Arch. Dermatol.* 1998; 134: 1431–1435.
[51] S Aktan, E Ozmen, B Sanli. Anxiety, depression and the nature of acne vulgaris in adolecents. *Int. J. Dermatol.* 2000; 39(5):354-7.
[52] J A Cotterill, W J Cuncliffe. Suicide in dermatological patients. *Br. J. Dermatology* 1997; 137(2):246-50.
[53] V Henkel, M Moehrenschager, U Hegerl, H J Moeller, J Ring, W I Worret. Screening for depression in adult acne vulgaris patients: tools for the dermatologist. *J. Cosmet. Dermatol.* 2002; 1(4):202-7.
[54] Rapp D et al. Anger and acne: implication for quality of life, patient satisfaction and clinical care. *British Journal of Dermatology.* 2004; 151:183-189.
[55] E Uhlenhake, B A Yentzer, S R Feldman. Acne vulgaris and depression: a retrospective examination. *J. Cosm. Dermatol.* 2010; 9(1);56-63.
[56] Panconesi. *Psychosomatic Dermatology in Clinics in Dermatology*, volume 4 no. 2. Stress and Skin Diseases: Psychosomatic Dermatology. Philadelphia: JB Lippincott, 1984. pg 135 -138.
[57] Fava GA, Tomba E. Increasing Psychological Well-Being and Resilience by Psychotherapeutic Methods. *Journal of Personality* 2009: 77:6, 1903-1934.
[58] Yi J, Vitalioano P, Smith R et al. The role of resiolience on psychological adjustment and physical health in patients with diabetes. *Br. J. Health Psychol.* 2008; 13: 311-325.
[59] Kristin Billaud Feragen, Ingela L Kvalem, Nchola Rumsey, Anne IH Borge The role of friendships and social acceptance in perceptions of appearance and emotional resilience in adolescents with and without a facial difference *Body Image* 2010 7; 271-279.
[60] Peterson C, Moier S, Seligman M. Learned helplessness: A Theory for the Age of Personal Control, 1996, OUP, USA.
[61] Koblenzer C. Psychodermatology of women. *Clin. Dermatol.* 1997; 15: 127-41.
[62] Brown BC, McKenna SP, Siddhi K, McGrouther DA, Bayat A. *J. Plast. Reconstr. Aesthet. Surg.* 2008 Sep;61(9):1049-58. The hidden cost of

skin scars: quality of life after skin scarring. Brown BC, McKenna SP, Solomon M, Wilburn J, McGrouther DA, Bayat A *Plast Reconstr Surg.* 2010 May;125(5):1439-49. The patient-reported impact of scars measure: development and validation.

[64] Brown BC, Moss TP, McGrouther DA, Bayat A. Skin scar preconceptions must be challenged: importance of self-perception in skin scarring. *J. Plast. Reconstr. Aesthet. Surg.* 2010 Jun;63(6):1022-9. Epub 2009 Jun 5 Sneddon J, Sneddon I. Acne excoriee: a protective device. *Clin. Exp. Dermatol.* 1983; 8: 65-8.

[66] Bach M, Bach D. Psychiatric and psychometric issues in acne excoriee. *Psychother. Psychosom.* 1993; 60: 207-10.

[67] Kent A, Drummond LM. Acne excoriee – a case report of treatment using habit reversal. *Clin. Exp. Dermatolol.* 1989; 14: 163-4.

[68] Gupta MA, Gupta AK. Olanzapine may be an effective adjunctive therapy in the management of acne excoriee: a case report. *J. Cutan. Med. Surg.* 2001; 5: 25-7.

[69] Philips K.A. The Broken Mirror: Understanding and Treating Body Dysmorphic Disorder, 2005, OUP, USA.

[70] Uzun O. *et al.* Body Dysmorphic Disorder in Patients with Acne. *Comprehensive Psychiatry.* 2003; 44:415-419.

[71] W P Bowe, J J Leyden, C E Crerand, B D Sarwer, D J Margolis. Body dysmorphic symptoms among patients with acne vulgaris. *J. Am. Acad. Dermatol.* 2007; 57(2):222-30.

[72] Phillips KA et al. A comparison of delusional and nondelusional body dysmorphic disorder in 100 cases. *Psychopharmacol. Bull.* 1994;30(2):179-86.

[73] Hull, SM, Cunliffe WJ, Huges BR. Treatment of the depressed and dysmorphophobic acne paient. *Clin. Exp. Dermatol.* 1991: 16: 210-211.

[74] Veale D. Cognitive-behavioural therapy for body dysmorphic disorder. *Advances in Psychiatric Treatment* 2001, 7: 125-132.

[75] *Mayo Clin. Proc.* 2011 Aug;86(8):792-800. Practical suicide-risk management for the busy primary care physician. McDowell AK, Lineberry TW, Bostwick JM.

[76] Palmer SC, Coyne JC. Screening for depression in medical care. Pitfalls, alternatives and revised priorities. *Journal of Psychosomatic Research.* 2003;54:279-287.

[77] Henkel V *et al.* Screening for depression in adult acne vulgaris patients: tools for the dermatologist. *Journal of Cosmetic Dermatology.* 2002; 1:202-207.

[78] Snyderman D, Rovner B. Mental Status Examination in Primary Care: A Review. *Am. Fam. Physician* 2009; 80: 809-14.
[79] *Acta Psychiatr. Scand.* 1983 Jun;67(6):361-70. The hospital anxiety and depression scale. Zigmond AS, Snaith RP.
[80] Barnes LE. *et al.* Quality of Life Measures for acne patients. *Dermatol. Clin.* 2012; 30:293-300.
[81] Nijsten T. Dermatology life quality index: time to move forward. *J. Invest. Dermatol.* 2012; 132:11-13.
[82] Rogers A, DeLong LK, Chen SC. Clinical meaning in skin-specific quality of life instruments: a comparison of the Dermatology Life Quality Index and Skindex banding systems. *Dermatol. Clin.* 2012; 30: 333-342.
[83] Wysowski D. Depression and Suicide in Patients Treated with Isotretinoin. *N. Engl. J. Med.* 2001; 344:460.
[84] Kellett SC, Gawkrodger DJ. A prospective study of the responsiveness of depression and suicidal ideation in acne patients to different phases of Isotretinoin therapy. *Eur. J. Dermatol.* 2005; 15: 484-8.
[85] Bremner JD. *et al.* Retinoic Acid and affective Disorders: The Evidence for an Association. *J. Clin. Psychiatry.* 2012; 73:37-50.

Chapter VII

Light Cautery in the Treatment of Closed Comedones

V. Bettoli, S. Zauli and A. Virgili
Section of Dermatology,
Department of Clinical and Experimental Medicine,
University of Ferrara, Italy

Abstract

Closed comedones are non inflammatory acne lesions which frequently precede inflammatory acne lesions. They consist on depositions of sebum surrounded by layers of horny cells and they can persist for a long time unless they are treated. Persistence of closed comedones may be responsible for reduced response to acne treatments and flare-up of inflammatory acne during oral isotretinoin assumption. Moreover, closed comedones, if not properly treated, are responsible for psychological distress in patients with acne; therefore their treatment is fundamental to improve quality of life.

Topical and systemic retinoids are the mainstay of their medical treatment, but although used for long periods of time they can be unsuccessful. Therefore their extraction is a mandatory procedure to obtain full clearance of acne.

Alternative treatments to eliminate closed comedones include cautery, surgery (physical extraction) and laser. Comparative studies matching different tecniques are not available in the literature.

The authors describe the techniques of light cautery in the treatment of close comedones and compare efficacy and tolerability of this procedure with the other aforementioned treatments.

Moreover they report their personal experience.

Introduction

Closed comedones, also called whiteheads, are non inflammatory acne lesions composed of depositions of sebum surrounded by layers of horny cells, without a direct external opening. They may not heal spontaneously and can persist for a long time unless they are treated [1].

Persistence of closed comedones may be responsible for reduced response to acne treatments. The use of oral isotretinoin may even result in a severe flare-up related to the presence of closed comedones [2], therefore their treatment is highly recommended, possibly before the beginning of the retinoid. Independently of the treatment used, to obtain the full clearance of acne and to maintain it, closed comedones must be eliminated. Furthermore, they can rupture and turn into large inflammatory acne lesions.

Moreover, closed comedones are disfiguring and difficult, sometimes impossible, to camouflage using make-up. They can be responsible for psychological distress in patients with acne; therefore their treatment is fundamental as it improves the patients' quality of life and self-esteem, and to decrease psychological morbitidity.

Unfortunately closed comedones are often unresponsive to both topical and systemic treatments. Topical retinoids have been successfully used for many years to treat non-inflammatory acne lesions, but sometimes they may have little or no effect, mostly on the larger whiteheads [3].

Alternative treatments to eliminate closed comedones include cautery, surgery (mechanical extraction) and laser [4]. Cautery, also called electrocautery, is effective, easily accessible and requires minimal training. It can be used in combination with topical or systemic therapy to maximize the therapeutic outcome [5].

The Procedure

Before begining the procedure, the skin is prepared for 1-2 hours with a 2-3 mm thick layer of the local anesthetic EMLA® cream (lidocaine 25 mg/g and prilocaine 25 mg/g) (Figure 1A) applied beneath a polyurethane, waterproof, transparent film (Figure 1B) [3, 6]. It is then removed with a dry swab. The use of EMLA® cream numbs the skin but it does not result in complete analgesia [6]. In literature some patients with too numerous and widespread lesions were treated under general anesthesia [7].

The skin must be pinched and pulled gently between the fingers or stretched to make deeper and smaller comedones more visible. It must be borne in mind that EMLA® cream produces a transient blanching of the skin, making visualization of the whiteheads difficult unless careful lighting and palpation are used [3]. Additionally, some whiteheads can become less palpable, probably due to the extra hydration of the skin created by the anaesthetic cream, reducing the difference in contours between normal and abnormal skin [8].

A cautery is a device that through a direct current produces temperatures up to 1200°C. Disposable or rechargeable devices are commercially available, the latter offer the possibility of changing the tip. Three different types of tip are available: fine, wide and long. Generally a fine tip is preferable for treatment of acne lesions.

The comedones are touched very gently in the center of their surface for less that 1 second with the cautery tip (Figure 1C). To produce little or no pain, the temperature of the cautery should be sufficient to just char paper towelling [5]. During the procedure the cautery tip should not be red in colour but grey or slightly orange [7]. The procedure takes 5-20 minutes depending on the number of lesions [3].

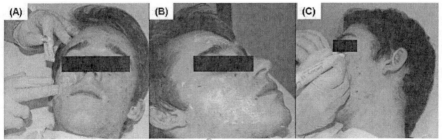

A. Application of a thick layer of EMLA® cream.
B. EMLA® cream beneath a polyurethane, waterproof and transparent film.
C. The cautery gentle touches the center of a comedone.

Figure 1. Light cautery technique.

After opening close comedones some authors pinch and pull the skin again between the thumb and index finger or use a dissecting forceps to make content extraction easier [6].

After each session an antibiotic cream should be applied on the treated area and it is advisable to use the same ointment twice daily until complete healing [6].

If correctly done, the treated lesions heal quickly in 4-7 days without any complication, in particular without scarring, [3]. Pigment changes rarely result from this treatment [3].

The procedure is in general well tolerated by the patients who are pleased with the results.

Long term results are good, but new comedones may form to replace those removed making additional sessions necessary. A topical retinoid should be applied to prevent the formation of new comedones.

If further sessions are needed, due to the presence of new closed comedones or to the impossibility of treating all the lesions in a single session because many of them are adjacent one to another, an interval of 1-2 weeks is necessary [6].

Literature Review

Light cautery has been shown to help patients with multiple closed comedones in four clinical studies [3, 6-8]. However it has been observed that it is less effective in severe cases with old and deep closed comedones larger than 3 mm in diameter [6].

Kaya et al. have used cautery also for the treatment of open comedones (blackheads) as extraction from a small pore is very difficult, and squeezing these lesions without previously widening them causes an important tissue trauma and pain. They applied a cautery point to the open comedones to widen their pores and facilitate the extraction [6].

Six patients with chloroacne, successfully treated with cautery following topical anaesthesia with EMLA® cream, are also reported in the literature [9].

The exact mechanism by which resolution occurs with cautery is unknown. Two theories have been suggested. The thermal damage produced by cautery stimulates the patients' own inflammatory reaction to induce distruction of the closed comedones. In alternative, or in addition, cautery may result in exteriorization of the lesion, providing a route for the content to discharge outside [3, 7].

Comparative studies matching cautery with mechanical extraction or laser do not exist in the literature.

Instead one study compared cautery with fulguration, obtained by a monopolar electrical current. This study reveals a significant difference in favour of cautery when treating closed comedones larger than 1 mm, whereas no significant difference between the two modalities have been observed in the treatment of the lesions of 1 mm or less. The cosmetic changes also differed very little between the two techniques [8]. Fulguration is a old technique that is no longer reported among physical treatments used in acne patients [5].

Authors' Experience

In the authors' personal experience light cautery is highly effective in reducing the number of closed comedones. The vast majority of the patients is willing to repeat the treatment and to suggest that other patients undergo it. Rarely the procedure is not well tolerated despite topical anesthesia.

In order to prevent S. aureus infection the authors advise the application of mupirocine, fusid acid or retapamulin for 10 days after cautery. The healing of the treated area occurs in a couple of weeks and, during this period of time, the patients can use camouflage.

The authors prefer to wait al least one month before repeating the treatment in order to allow complete healing of the previously treated area. Application of topical retinoids is suggested to prevent the formation of new closed comedones and to treat those that remain.

References

[1] Cunliffe, WJ; Holland, DB; Clark, SM; Stables, GI. Comedogenesis: some new aetiological, clinical and therapeutic strategies. *Br. J. Dermatol.*, 2000 142, 1084-1091.

[2] Bottomley, WW; Cunliffe, WJ. Severe flares of acne following isotretinoin: large closed comedones (macrocomedones) are a risk factor. *Acta Derm. Venereol.*, 1993 73, 74.

[3] Pepall, LM; Cosgrove, MP; Cunliffe, WJ. Ablation of whiteheads by cautery under topical anaesthesia. *Br. J. Dermatol.*, 1991 125, 256-259.
[4] Kaminsky, A. Less common methods to treat acne. *Dermatology*, 2003 206, 68-73.
[5] Dreno, B. Acne: physical treatment. *Clin. Dermatol.*, 2004 22, 429-433.
[6] Kaya, TI; Tursen, U; Kokturk, A; Ikizoglu, G. An effective extraction technique for the treatment of closed macrocomedones. *Dermatol. Surg.*, 2003 29, 741-744.
[7] Thomson, KF; Goulden, V; Sheehan-Dare, R; Cunliffe, WJ. Light cautery of macrocomedones under general anaesthesia. *Br. J. Dermatol.*, 1999 141, 595-596.
[8] Bottomley, WW; Yip, J; Knaggs, H; Cunliffe, WJ. Treatment of closed comedones-comparisons of fulguration with topical tretinoin and electrocautery with fulguration. *Dermatology*, 1993 186, 253-257.
[9] Yip, J; Peppall, L; Gawkrodger, DJ; Cunliffe, WJ. Light cautery and EMLA in the treatment of chloracne lesions. *Br. J. Dermatol.*, 1993 128, 313-316.

Index

A

abnormal differentiation of skin keratinocytes, ix, 69
abnormal keratinization, viii, 15, 72
academic performance, 109
acarbose, 78, 79, 87
access, 132
acid, 7, 9, 10, 11, 24, 25, 27, 28, 30, 33, 34, 37, 38, 45, 48, 53, 63, 73, 78, 90, 137, 151
acne vulgaris, vii, viii, x, 5, 7, 12, 13, 15, 16, 18, 23, 24, 30, 33, 34, 35, 36, 37, 38, 39, 43, 61, 62, 70, 81, 83, 85, 89, 99, 100, 101, 102, 103, 107, 117, 118, 123, 130, 140, 141, 143, 144
acquired immunity, 77
acromegaly, 73, 82
ACTH, 72, 75, 101
AD, 65, 66, 67, 83
additives, 3
adenosine, 95
adhesion, 105
adipose, 101
adipose tissue, 101
adjunctive therapy, 144
adjustment, xi, 108, 113, 125, 143

adolescents, vii, xi, 14, 31, 33, 34, 39, 71, 77, 107, 109, 110, 111, 118, 119, 126, 127, 128, 136, 141, 142, 143
adrenal gland, 75
adrenocorticotropic hormone, 72, 101
adulthood, vii, viii, 1, 5, 16, 32, 61, 141
adults, 32, 33, 78, 114, 122, 132
adverse effects, 26, 98, 121
adverse event, 26, 32, 35
aetiology, 19, 125
affective disorder, 137
Africa, 5, 11, 13
age, 5, 10, 16, 17, 43, 45, 71, 73, 91, 99, 118, 121, 134
aggressiveness, 92
agonist, 103
alcohol use, 132
alcohols, 51
aldehydes, 49
alkaloids, 49
aloe, 50
alopecia, 31, 39
alopecia areata, 31, 39
amenorrhea, 48, 105
amino acid(s), 30, 71
amyloid beta, 63
anaerobic bacteria, 4, 44
analgesic, 2
anatomy, viii, 1

Index

androgen(s), ix, x, 7, 22, 43, 45, 69, 70, 72, 73, 74, 75, 76, 79, 83, 84, 87, 89, 90, 123
anger, vii, 109, 110, 119, 123, 136
angina, 122
anorexia nervosa, 130
antagonism, 95
antibiotic, ix, 9, 10, 24, 26, 29, 42, 45, 46, 61, 91, 100, 150
antibiotic resistance, ix, 10, 29, 42, 61, 100
anti-cancer, 60, 68
antigen, 96, 97
anti-inflammatory agents, 47
anti-inflammatory drugs, 10
antimicrobial therapy, 36
antioxidant, ix, 42, 49, 51, 53, 57, 58
antipsychotic, 130
anxiety, vii, xi, 31, 39, 48, 108, 110, 115, 119, 125, 132, 134, 136, 145
anxiety disorder, xi, 108, 125, 136
apoptosis, 25, 30, 60, 67, 76
appetite, 2, 133
aptitude, 46
artery, 85
arthritis, 17
ASEAN, 47, 50, 62
Asian countries, 47
assessment, xi, 37, 39, 64, 108, 109, 122, 129, 130, 131, 133, 134, 135, 136, 138, 139, 140
assessment tools, 134, 139
asthma, 122
atopic dermatitis, 31, 39
atopic eczema, 122
attractant, 9
aversion, 124
avoidance, 121, 124, 125

bacteriostatic, 10, 11, 53, 79
bacterium, 20
bad habits, 31
basal layer, 98
base, 95
bed-wetting, 130
beneficial effect, 2, 13, 118
benefits, 23, 45, 47, 61
benzoyl peroxide, viii, 9, 10, 15, 34, 35, 36, 37, 38, 45, 51, 90
binding globulin, 81, 85
bioassay, 60
bioavailability, 71
biochemistry, 101
biofeedback, 113
biological activities, 50, 51, 63
biological media, 58
biologically active compounds, viii, 1, 10
biosynthesis, 73, 75
bipolar disorder, 138
birth control, 91
blood, 49, 64
body image, vii, 109, 115, 116, 117, 119, 120, 124, 130
body index, 31
body mass index (BMI), 72, 120
body weight, 58, 59, 137
bonding, 126
bone, 80
bone growth, 80
bradykinin, 59, 66
breast cancer, 60, 67, 80
bulimia, 130
bullying, 121
Burma, 51, 52
burn, 2
by-products, 3

B

bacillus, 43
bacteria, ix, 10, 13, 20, 26, 42, 44, 45, 46, 47, 49, 51, 54, 56, 57, 64, 65, 66
bacterial cells, 26
bacterial colonization, ix, 69
bacterial infection, viii, 8, 41

C

Ca^{2+}, 101
Cambodia, 52
cancer, 2, 23, 31, 60, 72, 86
candidates, ix, 42, 57
carbohydrate(s), ix, 70, 77

Index

carcinogenesis, 60
cascades, 33
causal relationship, 32
cell cycle, 25, 76
cell death, 67
cell differentiation, 25, 70, 75, 76, 97
cell line(s), 34, 35, 60, 61, 67, 68, 101
challenges, 115
cheese, 77
chemical, ix, 25, 27, 42, 49, 52, 53, 65, 118
chemical peel, 27, 118
chemical stability, 65
chemotaxis, 25, 26
chemotherapeutic agent, 60
chemotherapy, 60
childhood, 81, 109, 116, 130, 142
children, 5, 28, 78, 86, 107, 118, 122, 128, 142
cholera, 94
cholesterol, x, 70, 74, 94, 96
chromatography, 54, 64, 65
chronic diseases, 132
chronic illness, 119
circulation, 71, 80
civilization, 3, 81, 85
clarity, 138
classes, 96
classification, 4, 33
cleft lip, 127
cleft palate, 128
climate, 52
clinical assessment, 129
clinical depression, 31, 131, 132, 137
clinical trials, 30
cloning, 103
close relationships, 128
clothing, 124
cognition, 48, 135
cognitive therapy, 130
collagen, 48, 49, 63
colon, 59, 67
colon cancer, 60
colon carcinogenesis, 59
colonisation, 20
colonization, ix, 20, 46, 69, 72, 74

colorectal cancer, 60, 67
combination therapy, 25, 26, 38, 91
commercial, 51, 124
communication, xi, 108, 109, 113, 129
communication skills, xi, 108, 113, 129
community, 5, 48, 100, 119, 140
comorbidity, xi, 108, 132, 141
complement, 7
complications, 17
composition, 34, 81
compounds, ix, 11, 42, 51, 53, 55, 58, 60, 64, 66, 68
Concise, 13, 141
concordance, 109
conference, 12
conflict, 111
consciousness, 115
consensus, 109
constituents, 48, 49, 52, 53, 58, 61, 63
consulting, 17
consumers, 3
consumption, 22, 77, 78, 81, 86
contact dermatitis, 25, 27
contraceptives, 91
controlled trials, 35
controversial, 22, 28, 32, 43, 77
coping strategies, 110
correlation, x, 9, 58, 70, 72, 78, 91, 121, 122, 129
corticosteroids, 123
corticotropin, 143
cosmetic(s), ix, 3, 11, 14, 17, 42, 52, 116, 118, 119, 124, 142, 151
cost, 36, 143
cough, 2
CT, 65, 94
Cuba, 52
cultivation, 52
culture, 73, 94, 96, 103
curcumin, 47
cure, 31, 45, 48, 112, 124
cyclooxygenase, 49, 58
cytokines, viii, 1, 8, 9, 21, 44, 58, 74, 82, 93, 102
cytoplasm, 76

Index

cytotoxicity, 60

D

danger, 23
data analysis, 134
database, 137
defence, 35
deficiency, 72, 76, 83, 104
degradation, 53
dehydroepiandrosterone (DHEA), x, 70
delusions, 136
Department of Agriculture, 52
depression, vii, xi, 28, 30, 31, 39, 108, 119, 125, 132, 133, 134, 136, 139, 143, 144, 145
depressive symptoms, 31, 109, 120, 123, 127, 129, 132, 136, 137
derivatives, 11, 30, 45, 48, 50
dermatitis, 11, 26, 50, 91
dermatologist, vii, 33, 61, 131, 132, 135, 136, 143, 144
dermatology, xi, 2, 12, 14, 31, 37, 39, 64, 80, 100, 102, 108, 112, 121, 131, 132, 141, 142
dermatoses, 123, 140
dermis, 28, 102
despair, 110
destruction, 27, 28, 44
detection, 135
diabetes, viii, 15, 72, 122, 127, 143
diabetic patients, 78, 86
diagnostic criteria, 130
diarrhea, 48, 51
diet, 22, 34, 43, 77, 78, 81, 85, 86
digestion, 9
dihydrotestosterone (DHT), x, 43, 70
direct action, 70
disability, vii, 39, 112, 120, 126, 140
disappointment, 110
disclosure, 113, 126
discomfort, 32
disease progression, 90
diseases, vii, viii, 1, 10, 15, 31, 46, 48, 61, 81, 122, 142

disgust, 110, 113
disorder, viii, xi, 1, 10, 108, 125, 130, 133, 136, 138, 142, 144
dissatisfaction, 31, 128
distillation, 51
distress, 33, 127, 128, 129, 132
distribution, 31, 128
diuretic, 49
diversity, 11
DNA, 60, 76
DNA damage, 76
doctors, 111, 115, 123, 139
double bonds, 30
down-regulation, x, 70
drug reactions, 13
drug toxicity, 17
drugs, viii, 1, 2, 10, 11, 17, 25, 30, 36, 50, 61, 137
dysphoria, 117
dysthymia, 130

E

East Asia, ix, 42, 51, 63
eczema, 11, 48, 50, 112, 115, 123
edema, 59
editors, 62, 65
education, 109, 115, 119, 125, 130
Egypt, 3
electrocautery, 148, 152
electron, viii, 1, 6
ELISA, 58
emotion, 61, 123, 141
emotional distress, vii, 111, 127, 131
emotional problems, 122
emotional well-being, 129
empathy, xi, 108, 113
employment, 109
employment opportunities, 109
enamel, 6
endocrine, x, 70, 72, 77, 87, 103, 123, 143
endocrine disorders, x, 70
endocrine glands, 103
endonuclease, 60, 67
endothelial cells, 35, 103

energy, 30, 57, 92, 122, 133
England, 65, 129
enlargement, 34
environment, 44, 125
enzyme(s), x, 8, 9, 28, 44, 49, 57, 58, 60, 70, 72, 74, 75, 76, 84
epidemiologic, 33
epidermis, 4, 7, 27, 28, 43, 51, 73, 74, 83, 87, 92
epilepsy, viii, 15, 122
epithelia, 93, 103
epithelial cells, 92
epithelium, 44, 105
equilibrium, ix, 69
esophagitis, 29
estrogen, 43, 75, 91
ethanol, 53, 54
ethnic groups, 16
ethyl acetate, 54
etiology, viii, 1, 15, 31
evidence, ix, 2, 21, 22, 29, 33, 35, 64, 69, 72, 76, 77, 78, 102, 115, 123, 130, 137
evolution, 23, 32
excretion, x, 70, 73, 82, 100
exercise, 116
exposure, 9, 10, 22, 45, 60
extracellular matrix, 92, 104
extraction, xii, 53, 54, 65, 147, 148, 150, 151, 152
extracts, 2, 11, 13, 53, 54, 55, 56, 57, 60, 65, 66

F

families, 128
family conflict, 109
family members, 31
fat, 11, 77, 78
fatty acids, 20, 44, 74, 83, 104
FDA, 136
fear(s), 110, 125, 130, 135
feelings, 31, 107, 110, 113, 125, 136
fever, 48
fibroblasts, x, 49, 70, 76, 82, 92
flavonoids, 49, 50, 51, 53, 55, 57

fluid, 3
fluorescence, 30, 38
follicle(s), viii, ix, 4, 7, 19, 20, 41, 43, 44, 45, 46, 69, 72, 73, 74, 84, 92
food, 22, 77, 81, 136
formation, x, 3, 9, 10, 12, 20, 30, 42, 43, 49, 63, 70, 77, 90, 119, 150, 151
free radicals, 25, 26, 30, 53, 57
Freud, 111
friend support, 127
fruits, ix, 42, 51, 66
funding, 61
fungi, 47, 51

G

gel, 34, 35, 36, 37, 38, 54
gene expression, 21, 48
general anaesthesia, 152
general anesthesia, 149
genes, 21, 59, 73, 76, 82, 84, 101
genetic predisposition, 4
genetics, 43, 44
genome, 74, 83
genus, 14
Germany, 119
gland, x, 7, 19, 20, 22, 34, 43, 45, 46, 72, 73, 74, 75, 81, 82, 89, 90, 92, 97, 98, 99, 102, 104, 105, 123
glucocorticoid(s), 43, 72
glucose, 79, 85, 86, 87
glucose tolerance, 85, 87
glucose tolerance test, 85
glucoside, 50
GLUT4, 79
glycoside, 50
gonorrhea, 49
grades, 4
grading, 117, 118
Greece, 3
growth, ix, 11, 26, 34, 43, 44, 49, 60, 69, 70, 71, 72, 77, 79, 80, 81, 82, 83, 84, 85, 86, 87
growth factor, ix, 34, 43, 69, 71, 79, 80, 81, 82, 83, 84, 85, 86, 87

growth hormone, 72, 79, 80, 81, 82, 83, 84, 87
growth spurt, 81
guidance, 56, 62
guidelines, 28, 132
guilt, 110
guilty, 133

H

hair, 3, 9, 38, 43, 45, 73, 92
hair follicle, 3, 38, 43, 45, 73, 92
hairless, 22, 34
Hawaii, 52
headache, 2, 28
healing, 2, 48, 49, 51, 150, 151
health, viii, xi, 2, 3, 42, 50, 61, 80, 108, 122, 125, 132, 141
health care, 2, 50
heat shock protein, 103
height, 50
helplessness, 143
heme, 82
heme oxygenase, 82
hepatitis, 46
hepatocellular carcinoma, 67
hepatoma, 60, 85
herbal medicine, viii, 11, 41, 49, 62
herpes, 2
hexane, 54, 60
histamine, 51, 58, 59, 64, 66
history, 16, 62, 112, 130, 132, 136
HM, 64, 83
homeostasis, 79, 92
hormone(s), ix, 43, 44, 62, 69, 70, 71, 72, 76, 80, 81, 82, 85, 101, 104, 143
host, 4, 7, 74, 83
hostility, 119
human, vii, x, 2, 4, 9, 19, 21, 33, 35, 48, 49, 59, 60, 63, 64, 67, 70, 71, 73, 75, 76, 80, 82, 83, 84, 85, 87, 90, 92, 94, 95, 96, 97, 98, 99, 100, 101, 102, 103, 104, 105
human body, 73
human neutrophils, 9

human skin, x, 4, 70, 71, 80, 82, 83, 90, 92, 97, 98, 102, 105
hydrocarbons, 51
hydrogen, 49, 57
hydrogen peroxide, 49
hydroxyl, 58, 60
hygiene, 43
hyperandrogenism, 75, 76, 78
hyperglycaemia, ix, 70
hyperglycemia, 77
hyperinsulinemia, 76, 77, 78
hyperplasia, 22, 72
hypertension, 122
hypnosis, 111
hypnotherapy, 113
hypoglycemia, 79
hypothalamus, 70
hypothesis, 21, 76, 93, 123

I

iatrogenic, 17
ideal(s), 30, 53, 116
identity, 119
IL-8, viii, 1, 8, 9, 21, 44, 59, 74, 83, 103
image(s), vii, 95, 96, 98, 109, 111, 116, 117, 136, 140
image analysis, 98
imagery, 113
immune disorders, 3
immune response, 21, 58
immune system, 7, 20, 123
immunity, 143
immunomodulatory, 34
immunoreactivity, 92, 93
improvements, 119
in vitro, x, 49, 63, 64, 70, 71, 87, 93, 94, 95, 96, 99, 100, 101, 104
in vivo, 22, 34, 59, 63, 71, 87, 93, 95, 97, 101, 105
incidence, 5, 28, 29, 31, 72
India, 52
individuals, xi, 72, 107, 109, 116, 117, 121, 124, 129, 131
Indonesia, 52, 65

Index

induction, 58, 67, 76, 83, 84
industry(s), ix, 2, 14, 42, 52, 61, 116
infection, 10, 29, 51, 61, 91, 151
inferiority, 107, 110, 113
inflammation, viii, ix, 7, 9, 11, 15, 17, 20, 21, 22, 25, 44, 45, 46, 47, 52, 58, 59, 64, 66, 67, 69, 72, 74, 90, 92
inflammatory cells, 26
inflammatory disease, ix, 21, 69, 101
inflammatory mediators, 7, 123
ingredients, 3
inhibition, x, 25, 31, 34, 57, 59, 60, 71, 76, 89, 91, 94, 96, 98
inhibitor, 64, 79, 87
initiation, 33, 75, 90, 102, 118
injuries, 2, 51
innate immunity, 21
insecurity, 107
insomnia, 133
insulin, ix, 22, 34, 43, 67, 69, 71, 72, 73, 76, 77, 78, 79, 80, 81, 82, 83, 84, 85, 86, 87
insulin resistance, 22, 67, 72, 73, 76, 77, 78, 79, 85, 86
insulin sensitivity, 72, 77, 79, 81, 83
insulin signaling, 84
insulin-like growth factor-1, ix, 34, 69, 81, 82, 83, 87
integration, 119
integrin, 104
interference, 121
interferon, 83
interleukin-8, 21, 33
intervention, ix, 69, 112
investment, 116
irradiation, 30
irritability, 136
isolation, 17, 54, 115, 128
issues, 109, 144
Italy, 15, 31, 69, 147

J

Jamaica, 52
Java, 52
justification, 31

K

kaempferol, 49, 50
keratin, 3, 44
keratinocyte(s), ix, x, 8, 21, 33, 44, 49, 64, 69, 70, 74, 77, 83, 87, 92, 93, 101, 102, 103
kill, 57

L

lack of confidence, 123, 139
lactose, 77
lasers, 38, 46
later life, 116
lattices, 49
lead, 29, 58, 68, 72, 91, 110, 114, 117, 131
leadership, 126
learned helplessness, 129
leisure, 129, 134
leprosy, 48
lesions, viii, x, xii, 3, 4, 5, 7, 17, 18, 19, 20, 21, 23, 27, 31, 41, 46, 48, 51, 67, 70, 72, 74, 89, 90, 130, 147, 148, 149, 150, 151, 152
leukemia, 67
life quality, 145
life satisfaction, 117
light, xii, 20, 22, 30, 33, 38, 46, 62, 93, 136, 148, 151
lipases, 7, 8
lipid peroxidation, 58
lipids, x, 7, 28, 30, 89, 90, 93, 94, 95, 96, 97, 98, 104
lipolysis, 92, 101
liquid chromatography, 96
liver, 70, 71, 76
local anesthetic, 148
localization, 80, 82, 99
longitudinal study, 81
low risk, 132
lung cancer, 60
lupus, 48
luteinizing hormone, 75, 84

M

macrophages, 9
magazines, 124
majority, 42, 71, 102, 114, 115, 118, 129, 138, 151
malaria, 2
Malaysia, 52
man, 99
management, viii, xi, 12, 29, 32, 34, 35, 39, 61, 62, 80, 82, 99, 103, 108, 109, 112, 123, 125, 129, 140, 144
mass, 31, 64, 72, 119
mass spectrometry, 64
mast cells, 92
matrix, 7, 9
matrix metalloproteinase, 7
matter, 137
MB, 139
meat, 78, 86
median, 137
medical, viii, ix, xii, 12, 13, 31, 32, 42, 63, 109, 110, 111, 112, 126, 134, 139, 144, 147
medical care, 144
medical history, 32
medication, 44, 45, 61, 134
medicine, viii, ix, 1, 2, 12, 13, 42, 48, 60, 112, 113, 140
melanocortin receptors, x, 89, 92
melanocyte stimulating hormone, 92, 101, 102, 103, 104
melting, 54
membranes, 7, 95
mental health, xi, 17, 31, 33, 39, 108, 122, 131, 132, 136, 137
mental health professionals, 136
mental illness, 132
messenger ribonucleic acid, 84
messenger RNA, 76
Metabolic, 104
metabolic syndrome, 85
metabolism, 76, 78, 83, 101
metabolites, 74
metabolized, 27, 30

metformin, x, 70, 78, 79, 87
mice, x, 22, 34, 38, 59, 89, 92, 93, 95, 96, 97, 98, 102
microbiota, 4
microorganisms, 13, 56
microRNA, 60
migration, 64
mitochondria, 30, 67
mitogen, 80, 82
MMP, 9
model system, 97
modelling, 115
models, 30, 120, 139
modern society, 116
modifications, x, 31, 70
molecular oxygen, 30
molecular weight, 9
molecules, 8
monocyte chemoattractant protein, 59
mood states, 119
morbidity, viii, xi, 32, 107, 109, 110, 116, 124, 132, 133, 134, 135, 138, 140
morphology, viii, 1
MR, 63, 85
mRNA, 21, 59, 67, 79, 87, 103
mucous membrane, 10
multidimensional, 116
musculoskeletal, 17
mutations, 13, 72
myoblasts, 80
myocardial infarction, 58, 66

N

nail biting, 130
natural compound, 57
necrosis, 27, 30
negative effects, 109, 128
negative emotions, 110
negativity, 125
neglect, 136
nervous system, 143
Netherlands, 14
neuropeptides, x, 89, 92, 103, 123
neutral, 94, 96, 131

neutral lipids, 96
neutrophil chemotactic factors, 44
neutrophils, 9
New Zealand, 5
Nigeria, 5
nightmares, 130
Nile, 94, 96, 104
nitric oxide, 58, 59
nitric oxide synthase, 59
nodules, 4, 5, 16, 17, 18, 19, 23, 28, 42, 48, 72
North America, 35
nuclear receptors, 77
nucleus, 76
nurses, 118
nutraceutical, 51
nutrition, 71

O

obesity, 85
obsessive-compulsive disorder, 125, 130
obstruction, viii, 4, 7, 15, 44, 45, 72
occlusion, 20
oil, 3, 11, 47, 49, 51, 64
oligomenorrhea, 105
oligomers, 63
optimism, 126
oral antibiotic(s), 25
organ, 3, 7, 70, 73
organelles, 30
organism, 8, 58
outpatient(s), 6, 32, 117, 122, 140
ovaries, 84
overproduction, viii, 41
oxidation, 30, 47, 53
oxidative damage, 64
oxidative stress, 77, 92
oxygen, 25, 26, 30, 57

P

pain, 51, 58, 117, 122, 149, 150
palate, 127
palpation, 149
Panama, 52
parallel, 85
parent pro-opiomelanocortin (POMC), x, 89
parents, 107, 114, 130
pathogenesis, viii, ix, 1, 7, 8, 9, 15, 19, 20, 21, 22, 43, 69, 72, 75, 81, 85, 90, 91, 99, 103, 109, 143
pathogens, 10
pathology, x, 22, 33, 89
pathophysiology, viii, ix, 7, 15, 69, 123
pathways, x, 21, 25, 70, 90, 91
patient care, 112
pattern recognition, 9
PCR, 59
peer relationship, 109
peptide(s), 7, 70, 93, 101, 102, 104
perfectionism, 117, 128, 136
peripheral blood mononuclear cell, 83
permeability, 7
peroxidation, 58
peroxide, 9, 24, 35, 36, 37, 45
personal hygiene, 125
personal qualities, 128
personal relations, 129, 134
personal relationship, 129, 134
personality, 110, 111, 116, 121, 126, 130, 141
personality disorder, 130
personality factors, 126
personality type, 111, 121
pessimism, 129
phagocytic cells, 57
pharmaceutical, 2, 3, 11, 48, 61, 112
pharmacology, 37, 99
phenolic compounds, 49, 53, 55, 57
phenotype, 34
Philadelphia, 143
Philippines, 52
phobia, 130
phosphate, 35, 36, 37
phosphorylation, 76
photographs, 124
photosensitivity, 10, 29, 45, 91
photosensitizers, 30

physical attractiveness, 118
physical health, 143
physical therapy, 130
physical treatments, 139, 151
physicians, 26, 30, 123, 129
physiology, 73, 78, 87, 100
PI3K, 76, 77
pigmentation, 92, 98, 101
pilot study, 85, 87, 140, 141
pioglitazone, 78
pituitary gland, 70, 93
placebo, 25, 26, 32, 34, 35, 138
plants, 2, 11, 13, 14, 46, 50, 51, 53, 57, 62, 64, 65, 66
plasma membrane, 30
plausibility, 137
polar, 53
polarity, 54
polycystic ovarian syndrome, 78
polymorphism(s), 72, 80, 81
polypeptides, 71
polyphenols, 11
polysaccharide(s), 11, 66
polyurethane, 149
poor relationships, 130
population, 9, 30, 33, 42, 115, 126, 131, 133, 142
porphyrins, 30
positive correlation, 75
precipitation, 55
pregnancy, 28, 45, 116
preparation, 53, 65
prevention, 58, 77, 90, 98, 112
principles, 30, 38
producers, 3
professionals, 125
progesterone, 43, 72, 91
pro-inflammatory, viii, 1, 8, 21, 58
proliferation, viii, 7, 15, 46, 64, 71, 74, 76, 83, 87, 90, 93, 99
proliferation of Propionibacterium acnes, viii, 15
promoter, 71
prostaglandins, 49
prostate cancer, 79, 87
protection, 3, 29, 49
protein synthesis, 26
proteins, 7, 9, 26, 30, 44, 60, 71, 73, 80, 82, 84, 104
psoriasis, 3, 31, 39, 48, 112, 122, 123
psychiatric diagnosis, 130
psychiatric disorders, xi, 108, 133, 138
psychiatric illness, 136
psychiatric morbidity, 31, 133
psychiatric side effects, 32, 137
psychiatrist, 112, 136
psychological association, 129
psychological distress, xii, 17, 31, 90, 147, 148
psychological health, 109, 124
psychological problems, 17
psychological processes, 31
psychological well-being, 31, 126, 127, 128
psychology, 110
psychopathology, 32, 39, 100, 110, 111, 115, 117, 130, 136, 138
psychosocial dysfunction, 124
psychosocial factors, 112
psychosomatic, viii, xi, 108, 112, 113, 123, 129, 138, 139
psychosomatic approach, xi, 108, 112, 113, 129, 138, 139
psychotherapy, 111, 112, 113, 130
pubertal development, 81
puberty, ix, 4, 5, 17, 43, 69, 72, 76, 81, 83, 114, 116
Puerto Rico, 52

Q

qualifications, 113
quality of life, xi, xii, 18, 39, 42, 90, 108, 109, 112, 115, 116, 118, 121, 122, 126, 129, 132, 134, 137, 138, 139, 141, 142, 143, 144, 145, 147, 148
quercetin, 53
questionnaire, 32, 34, 39, 112, 116, 119, 121, 122
quinone, 66

Index

R

radar, 135
radiation, 22, 34
radicals, 49, 57
rash, 50
rating scale, 4
RE, 35
reactions, 30
reactive oxygen, 30, 44, 48, 58
reactivity, 93
reading, 99
receptors, x, 7, 9, 20, 21, 25, 33, 43, 44, 59, 73, 74, 83, 89, 92, 105
recognition, 20, 140
recommendations, 22, 29, 99
recovery, 56
recreational, 124
recurrence, 61
regeneration, 105
regression, 31, 117
regression analysis, 117
regression model, 31
rehabilitation, 112
relatives, 121
relaxation, xi, 108, 111, 123
relevance, 2, 98
reliability, 55
repair, 76
repression, 76
repulsion, 92, 93
researchers, ix, 3, 42
residues, 7
resilience, xi, 107, 109, 126, 127, 132, 143
resistance, 10, 12, 13, 26, 29, 34, 36, 45, 46, 62, 76, 87, 91, 92, 100
resolution, 7, 16, 150
resources, 61, 127
response, xii, 4, 7, 8, 9, 44, 71, 73, 77, 79, 81, 83, 87, 92, 99, 101, 113, 123, 137, 147, 148
responsiveness, 137, 145
reticulum, 30
reversal training, xi, 108, 130
RH, 34

rhizome, 46, 47
rights, 141
risk(s), xi, 10, 28, 29, 31, 32, 34, 61, 80, 85, 91, 107, 109, 127, 128, 131, 132, 133, 135, 136, 138, 144, 151
risk factors, xi, 107, 109, 128, 132
risk management, 144
RNAs, 102
rodents, 93
romantic relationship, 31
roots, 10, 11, 60
Rosenberg Self-Esteem Scale, 117, 142
rosiglitazone, 79, 87

S

sadness, 110
safety, 3, 35, 37, 38
Salmonella, 57
salts, 79
scabies, 2
scaling, 91, 129
schema, 38, 118
school(ing), 5, 111, 115, 121, 123, 126, 130, 134
scope, 11
scotoma, 135
scrotal, 76
sebum, viii, ix, x, xii, 3, 7, 8, 15, 18, 20, 22, 34, 41, 43, 44, 45, 46, 69, 73, 74, 77, 82, 89, 90, 91, 93, 95, 96, 97, 98, 100, 104, 147, 148
sebum production, viii, ix, x, 7, 15, 18, 20, 22, 44, 45, 46, 69, 77, 89, 90, 93, 96, 97, 98
secrete, viii, 1, 7, 8, 9, 44, 97
secretion, ix, x, 4, 7, 21, 23, 34, 43, 69, 70, 71, 74, 75, 76, 81, 85, 89, 90, 91, 93, 95, 97, 98
selectivity, 30
self esteem, 109, 115, 118, 126, 128
self-assessment, 129, 133
self-confidence, 31, 115
self-consciousness, xi, 30, 107, 109, 110
self-efficacy, 126

self-esteem, vii, xi, 30, 31, 42, 61, 62, 80, 107, 109, 115, 116, 119, 123, 124, 126, 148
self-image, xi, 30, 31, 107, 109, 119, 130, 137
self-perceptions, 127
self-view, 127
self-worth, 31, 119, 120
senescence, 48
sensitivity, 72, 75, 116, 128, 133, 141
sensors, 20
serotonin, 58, 59, 66
serum, x, 34, 70, 71, 72, 74, 75, 77, 78, 79, 81, 82, 86, 87
settlements, 2
sex, 45, 71, 81, 85, 134
sexual activity, 92
sexuality, 116
shame, 141
shape, 117
showing, 115, 116
shyness, 115
sialic acid, 7
side effects, viii, ix, 1, 10, 23, 27, 28, 29, 42, 45, 46, 91, 137
signalling, ix, 21, 69, 72, 73, 76, 78
signs, 17, 132, 135
silica, 54
Singapore, 5
sinuses, 17
skin cancer, 3, 39
skin diseases, 3, 13, 18, 23, 34, 39, 49, 50, 112, 122, 123, 127, 142
sleep deprivation, 123
sleep disturbance, 133
social acceptance, 127, 128, 143
social consequences, 141
social events, 123, 124
social impairment, vii, 33
social interactions, 31
social phobia, xi, 108, 125, 130
social relationships, 116
social support, 110
social withdrawal, 109, 123, 131
solution, 29, 35, 36

solvents, 53
South Africa, 5, 11, 12, 14
South America, 49, 50, 52
Southeast Asia, 52
SP, 66, 79, 143, 144
Spain, 29
species, 10, 11, 30, 44, 48, 58, 61, 83
speech, 136
Sri Lanka, 52
SS, 61, 62, 63, 68
stability, 13, 54
standard deviation, 56
standardization, 56, 64, 65
state(s), 3, 52, 91, 115, 119, 125, 130
steroids, 50, 78
stigma, 114, 115, 129, 141
stimulation, 22, 75, 81, 84, 103
stomach, 2
storage, 54, 55
stress, xi, 77, 92, 101, 108, 110, 115, 117, 123, 130, 132
stress response, 92
structural protein, 44
structure, 25
subgroups, 122
SUbjective Discomfort Scores (SUDS), xi, 108, 132
suicidal behavior, 38
suicidal ideation, vii, 17, 31, 39, 113, 123, 136, 139, 145
suicide, vii, xi, 28, 32, 42, 108, 123, 131, 132, 136, 144
suicide attempts, vii, 123, 136
suicide rate, 137
sulfate, 81
sweat, 92
Sweden, 23
swelling, 46, 58
symptoms, 17, 34, 109, 119, 130, 133, 134, 137, 144
syndrome, 72, 75, 79, 81, 85, 86, 87
synthesis, x, 23, 48, 63, 70, 73, 74, 75, 76, 79, 82, 93, 95, 96, 97, 104

Index

T

tannins, ix, 42, 49, 51, 53, 55, 57
target, 44, 45, 67, 77, 79, 90, 101
techniques, xii, 110, 113, 148, 151
technology, 12, 14
teenage girls, 78, 86
teens, 114
temperature, 3, 54, 55, 149
testing, 54, 71
testis, 84
testosterone, x, 43, 44, 70, 74, 75, 76, 79, 83, 87, 93, 99, 104
tetracyclines, 29
textbook, 80
Thailand, 41, 47, 50, 51, 52, 55, 62, 65
therapeutic agents, xi, 90
therapeutic relationship, 131
therapeutics, 11
therapy, viii, x, xi, 9, 15, 22, 23, 25, 26, 27, 28, 29, 31, 33, 36, 38, 39, 46, 62, 79, 87, 89, 91, 96, 97, 98, 99, 108, 109, 111, 112, 130, 131, 136, 137, 138, 139, 140, 144, 145, 148
thermoregulation, 93
thoughts, 42, 113, 117, 125, 133
time frame, 109
tissue, 7, 44, 49, 66, 71, 74, 150
TLR, 25
TLR2, 9, 21
TLR4, 21
TNF, 8, 9, 21, 58
TNF-α, 21, 58
topical antibiotics, 26, 27, 118
toxin, 94
training, xi, 108, 113, 118, 123, 139, 148
traits, 92, 119
transcription, 21, 71, 73, 85
transcription factors, 21, 73
transmission, viii, 1
transmission electron micrographs, viii, 1
trauma, 107, 150
tremor, 136
trial, 11, 34, 35, 36, 37, 52, 85, 100, 119, 130, 138

triglycerides, 20, 34, 44, 74, 94, 95, 96
tuberculosis, 57
tumor, viii, 1, 8, 9, 47, 59, 60, 74, 101, 102
tumor necrosis factor, viii, 1, 8, 9, 59, 74, 101, 102
Turkey, 122
turnover, 27
type 2 diabetes, 79
tyrosine, 71

U

ulcer, 51
uniform, 139
United Kingdom (UK), 5, 107, 134
United States (USA), 12, 52, 78, 80, 82, 137, 143, 144
urinary tract, 49
UV, 22, 34, 93
UV irradiation, 34
UV light, 22
UV radiation, 23

V

Valencia, 102
validation, 55, 56, 144
vancomycin, 57, 66
variables, 119, 121, 127, 128, 139
variations, x, 70, 72
Vietnam, 52
visualization, 149
vitamin A, 25, 45, 137
vitamin D, 23
vomiting, 130
vulnerability, 112

W

water, 29, 92, 93
web, 115
weight loss, 22
well-being, 132
withdrawal, 139

workers, viii
World Health Organisation (WHO), 47, 62, 119, 133
World War I, 51
worldwide, 2, 18, 51, 90
wound healing, 64, 105

X

xanthones, ix, 42, 51, 58, 59, 60, 65, 66, 67
xenografts, 105

Y

yield, 51, 53, 54
young adults, 32, 85, 115
young people, viii, 31, 39
young women, 28

Z

zinc, x, 70, 78, 79, 87